BARRIERS AND FACILITATORS TO QUALITY HEALTH CARE

Spring 1975

BArriErs AND FACILITATOrs TO QUALITY HEALTH CArE

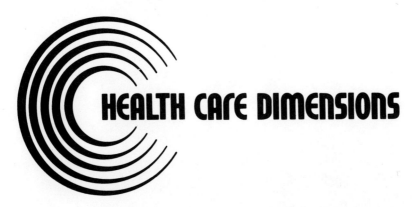

HEALTH CArE DIMENSIONS

Madeleine Leininger, R.N., Ph.D./Editor

Dean and Professor of Nursing and
Adjunct Professor of Anthropology
College of Nursing and Department of Anthropology
University of Utah, Salt Lake City, Utah

F. A. Davis Company, Philadelphia, Pa.

Library of Congress Cataloging in Publication Data

Leininger, Madeleine M
  Barriers and facilitators to quality health care.

  (Health care dimensions; Spring 1975)
  Includes bibliographies and index.
  1. Medical care—United States. 2. Medical personnel—United
States. 3. Medical policy—United States. 4. Nurses and nursing—
United States. I. Title. [DNLM: 1. Quality of health care. W1
HE299D / W84 B275]
RA395.A3L44   362.1'0973   74-32087
ISBN 0-8036-5526-6

Preface

The focus of this second issue of Health Care Dimensions, *Barriers and Facilitators to Quality Health Care,* follows logically from the first issue (Fall 1974) that dealt with several broad health care issues examined from a variety of perspectives. In this issue, several nationally known authors from various disciplines have addressed significant trends, barriers, and facilitating factors in health care delivery based upon their direct experiences. Their informative discussions support our major theme of "Let's share and discuss together."

Health care delivery in the United States is being altered in varying degrees in different parts of the country. There is a general optimism about changing health care patterns to make services more economical, comprehensive, satisfying, and accessible than ever before. Quality care at a reasonable cost is the dominant goal, spurring some of our most creative health care planners and designers into action.

Before positive and significant changes can be made, health care planners, designers, and implementors must be aware of existing facilitators and barriers to quality health care in our present system. Ideal plans must be made explicit, tested, and brought into close relationship with empirical realities. These are two important ideas in this second issue.

In the process of discovering barriers and facilitators to quality health care, new conceptual frameworks and models emerge which can help change health care delivery systems. These models should be designed to accomodate new types of health practitioners and new educational programs with respect to diverse cultural groups and sociopolitical interests in our society.

Our present health systems are generally large, stratified, complex and bureaucratized, and so we must take vigorous measures to reduce their complexity and make them as human as possible. We need to alter the dominant emphases in our health care systems from the present focus on *sickness and restoration* to that of *wellness and health maintenance.* Helping individuals and groups attain and maintain a desired health state is a major challenge for health care practices of tomorrow.

Another barrier to quality health care is the present emphasis on the special health needs and problems of *each individual.* While this highly individualized focus has humanistic value, we should also be concerned about the specific health needs and problems of community groups and special populations. Such an approach is actually anthropological, in that it involves understanding the daily life practices of designated groups of people. This community or population approach to health care delivery has barely been used in our society, even though its long and short range benefits seem self-evident. It is enormously valuable in preventing widespread illnesses.

It is also my view that we must vigorously study, synthesize, and use relevant available knowledge about the differing health maintenance styles and health care seeking behaviors among groups of people as we develop new health care delivery services. Presently we have considerable knowledge about medical sciences, but very meager knowledge about diverse health maintenance styles among different cultural and community groups. Such knowledge is essential in meeting health care needs. Accordingly, we need to consider how to facilitate active use of ideas and research findings from social and behavioral scientists and humanists as they relate to health care in order to attain a holistic approach to man's health needs. At present, such an integration is very limited.

An encouraging new direction being taken is the more adequate distribution and utilization of available health care talent. Involving "urbanized" health professionals in rural health care service is a major concern. Some rural communities are only beginning to receive the benefits of new types of health care services. Facilitation of the *best* utilization of various health professionals and semi-professionals according to their educational preparation and experience is a recent challenge. Full utilization of the talents of nurses, pharmacists, social workers, occupational therapists, and many other professionals in addition to physicians is a tremendous challenge and a goal yet to be achieved in most areas of the United States. Most encouraging is the fact that nursing, the largest health professional group, is becoming more active than ever before in asserting its social and professional responsibilities. Nurse-midwives, clinical nurse specialists, and clinical generalists are becoming more visible and active in their role of professional accountability. How other disciplines assert their social responsibilities will be of interest as well as how these different health disciplines will orchestrate their endeavors. Optimal manpower utilization involves the greatest barriers, yet has the greatest potential for facilitating quality health care delivery.

These and other barriers and facilitators to health care are considered by the contributors to this issue. The ideas presented here can serve as valuable discussion topics for students, community groups, and national legislation groups interested in health care as well as for health practitioners and designers of new modes of health care delivery in the United States and perhaps in other societies. Our discussions are intended to stimulate and encourage our readers to examine additional barriers and facilitators to health care from their own local, regional, and national perspectives.

This issue would not have been possible without the continued support and interest of the staff of the F. A. Davis Company. In addition, Phyllis Clark of the University of Utah provided important secretarial assistance essential to bringing this second issue into existance. I am grateful to her and to our editorial advisory board members who recruited excellent contributors for this issue. Our next issue will focus on multicultural health care delivery issues.

Madeleine Leininger

Editorial Advisory Board

Rozella Schlotfeldt, R.N., Ph.D.
    Professor of Nursing, School of Nursing
    Case Western Reserve University, Cleveland, Ohio

Special Consultants

Sheldon Rovin, D.D.S.
    Dean, School of Dentistry
    University of Washington, Seattle, Washington

Donald Sorby, Ph.D.
    Professor of Pharmacy, College of Pharmacy
    University of Washington, Seattle, Washington

Minnie Walton, M.S.
    Professor of Nursing, College of Nursing
    University of Utah, Salt Lake City, Utah

Donald Langsley, M.D.
    Professor and Chairman of Psychiatry
    University of California, Davis Campus
    Sacramento, California

Contributors

John H. Bryant, M.D.
    Director, School of Public Health
    Associate Dean of the Faculty of Medicine
    Columbia University, New York, New York

Loretta C. Ford, R.N., Ed.D., F.A.A.N.
    Dean and Professor of Nursing
    School of Nursing
    University of Rochester, Rochester, New York

Charles H. Goldsmith, Ph.D.
    Associate Professor, Department of Clinical Epidemiology and Biostatistics
    and Department of Applied Mathematics
    McMaster University, Hamilton, Ontario, Canada

Merwyn R. Greenlick, Ph.D.
    Director of the Health Services Research Center
    Kaiser Foundation Hospitals, Portland, Oregon

Brenda C. Hackett, B.A.
    Research Associate, Department of Clinical Epidemiology and Biostatistics
    McMaster University, Hamilton, Ontario, Canada

Nancy S. Keller, R.N., Ph.D.
    Nursing Care and Consultation, Ltd.
    Tucson, Arizona

Dorothy J. Kergin, R.N., M.P.H., Ph.D.
    Associate Dean of Health Sciences (Nursing), School of Nursing
    McMaster University, Hamilton, Ontario, Canada

Madeleine Leininger, R.N., Ph.D., F.A.A.N.
    Dean and Professor of Nursing and Adjunct Professor of Anthropology
    College of Nursing and Department of Anthropology
    University of Utah, Salt Lake City, Utah

James J. McCormack, Ph.D.
    Executive Vice President
    Areawide and Local Planning for Health Action, Inc. (ALPHA)
    Syracuse, New York

Peter M. Milgrom, D.D.S.
    Chairman, Community Dentistry
    University of Washington, Seattle, Washington

William A. M. Russell, M.D., C.C.F.P.(C)
    Active Staff Physician, West Lincoln Memorial Hospital
    Hamilton, Ontario, Canada

Ernest W. Saward, Ph.D.
    Professor of Social Medicine
    School of Medicine and Dentistry
    University of Rochester, Rochester, New York

Walter O. Spitzer, M.D., M.P.H.
    Associate Professor, Department of Clinical Epidemiology and Biostatistics
    and Department of Family Medicine
    McMaster University, Hamilton, Ontario, Canada

May A. Yoshida, R.N., M.N.
    Associate Professor, School of Nursing
    McMaster University, Hamilton, Ontario, Canada

Contents

BARRIERS AND FACILITATORS TO QUALITY HEALTH CARE

Reflections on the Past Decade in Health Manpower

LORETTA C. FORD, R.N., Ed.D.

During the past decade, the nation and the health care industry have viewed with rising alarm the warnings of a "health manpower crisis." Conditioned by the events of World War II to think in terms of shortages of health personnel, the public and its legislators, eager to avert another crisis, have supported the emergence of a variety of differently trained health workers. Health professionals, encouraged by the financial backing of government and other sources, picked up the gauntlet and engaged in the proliferation of new categories of personnel. By equating professional "needs" with health and illness "needs," programs designed to supply additional manpower often evolved from a profession's own image, thereby adjusting to the requirements of the profession. The implicit assumption was, "What's good for the provider is good for the consumer and vice versa" (a statement analgous to one made by the President of General Motors, Charles E. Wilson, who said, "What is good for the country is good for General Motors and vice versa").

Today the supply and demand aspects of health manpower present quite a different picture. The concern about numbers of health personnel has given way to concern about the quality of care, the cost of health care delivery, and priorities in health care need goals. Consequently, the declaration of a national health policy is considered paramount to future health manpower planning.

This chapter examines changes in health manpower supply, need, and demand during the past decade. It reviews the major developments in the 1960s, offers reflections on their impact and implications, and raises issues concerning the preparation, distribution, utilization, and evaluation of health manpower in the future. Specific emphasis is placed on the contributions and potentials of nursing.

Throughout the 1960s, great energy was expended on seeking solutions to manpower problems. Commissions and committees[5,16,50,54,55,73,75] were appointed to study needs and issues. Government bureaus were organized. Demonstration projects and training programs were initiated.[8,21,35,42,47,52,72,78,79] The error which

1

arose from a concentration on provider roles was compounded by a lack of communication among health professionals. This approach has not been successful in meeting the health care delivery demands, and high costs have inescapably resulted.

Evaluative research was conducted on programs and their products.[37] A plethora of data was generated in hundreds of published and unpublished reports (see References). Miller and Ferber[53] comprehensively reviewed the major studies on health manpower undertaken during the 1960s. Among those reviewed are: The 1959 Surgeon General's Consultant Group on Medical Education (the Bane Committee); the 1963 Surgeon General's Consultant Group on Nursing; the President's Commission on Health Disease, Cancer and Stroke (the 1964 DeBakey Commission); the 1966 National Commission on Community Health Services; the National Advisory Committee on Health Manpower (1967); and the Secretary's Committee on Hospital Effectiveness (1962). The consensus of these reports is that the prominent determinants of the manpower explosion are related to: (1) cyclic reactions accelerated by medical research which advanced medical knowledge and engendered specialization, thereby further extending medical research; (2) social and political forces that enlarged the scope of civil rights to include health care for all people and jettisoned health issues into the political arena; (3) technological advances made during the World War II, Korean, and Viet Nam conflicts which increased the demand for a host of allies health workers and offered a ready supply of personnel trained on battle fronts; and (4) at the end of the decade, the legislation for Medicare and Medicaid that called national attention to the overburdened and increasingly expensive health care delivery system (or nonsystem or conglomerate of subsystems, if one wishes to attempt classifying the variety of offerings).

Other publications focused upon the shortages in manpower and recommended increasing numbers of personnel in the standard health occupations, primarily medicine and nursing. It is interesting to review a sampling of the data generated from these writings:

1) Three and one-half million people were estimated to have been employed in the health industry (a tenfold increase since 1900).[60]

2) Seventy per cent of the nonphysician group were women in 30 to 120 occupational categories.[62]

3) Eighty billion dollars or 7.6 per cent of the national budget was spent annually on health care.[77]

4) Hospital employees numbered about 2.5 million.[60]

5) The number of hospital personnel increased 20 per cent between 1966 and 1969.[12]

6) Clinical services of hospitals were used by 2,285 health occupational programs. Almost 40 per cent of these sites were activated in two years (1967 to 1969).[12]

7) Of the 54,359 medical house officers, 18,436 were foreign medical graduates. Twelve thousand foreign medical graduates were licensed to practice in the United States.[27]

8) Six thousand allied health programs have been inaugurated.[4]

9) Physicians' assistants numbered about 1,000.[61]

10) A health manpower sourcebook[60] identified 125 different primary occupational titles and about 250 specialty or secondary occupational designations.

During this hectic period, nursing also generated some interesting data from its educational programs and practice. By 1972,[58]

1) Over 2 million (of the 3.5 million health workers) were in the occupation of nursing; 778,470 were registered nurses.

2) Slightly more than one-half the number of registered nurses were employed in hospitals.[31]

3) Balances in nursing education programs and enrollment were changing slowly to transfer more nursing education from hospital controlled schools to institutions of higher education. Of the 51,784 students who graduated in 1972, 41.7 per cent were from diploma programs; this is one-half the number in 1962. The number of baccalaureate programs increased 34 per cent, and the number of associate degree increased 23.8 per cent during the academic years 1970-71 and 1971-72.[32] According to 1972 statistics, there were 542 hospital controlled diploma programs, 528 associate degree (junior college-type programs) and 279 baccalaureate nursing programs.[33]

4) It is estimated there are approximately 2,000 nurses prepared for expanded role functions.

5) Attention to the qualitative shortages and maldistribution of certain types of nurses, such as clinical specialists, teachers, researchers, and statesmen, has taken precedence over concern about the total number of nursing personnel.

Examples of past efforts to avert the health manpower crisis abound.[2,6,13,34] A perusal of specific titles, goals, content, length, and admission requirements of programs that prepared new health workers is revealing. The titles, sponsorship, and purpose reveal the explicit purpose of bringing relief to the physician and extending his skills through task delegation to lesser prepared people by (1) the training of new physician-support personnel and (2) the extention of the traditional roles of currently available medical personnel to include tasks which can be safely delegated by the physician.[5] Physician's assistants and a host of other workers with many differing titles and specialties came into vogue as physician extenders.[42] While these allied health workers were prepared for a myriad of functions, there emerged a need for preparing health workers for ambulatory care.[17,19,39,54]

As social concern for the right of all people to health care grew, specific efforts to bring health services to deprived populations moved ambulatory care into the limelight. (Expansion of allied personnel in inpatient services preceded that in outpatient services. Technicians for the operating room, respiratory care, and a host of other specialities developed. Nurses expanded their roles in coronary and intensive care units and in midwifery in the hospital setting.) In ambulatory care, allied health personnel became visible to the public in a growing health care delivery concept—the neighborhood health center. The broad social goal of comprehensive personal health care for all people was articulated by social activists, politicians, and health professionals.[34,55,66,80] Neighborhood health centers and other newly established community services offered promising mechanisms to make health care accessible and available to certain segments of the population.

Staffing these new centers required unique organizational patterns and role changes for personnel. Changes generally emanated from studies of tasks which professionals performed.[2,7,37] Formulations of the needs of consumers or comprehensive health care delivery systems were noticeably lacking. Thus, new roles for technical and professional workers were graven images of traditional roles, growing extensive appendages to an already encumbered hierarchial, bureaucratic health care system.

New health workers were trained, as were their predecessors, in isolation from each other. Separate curriculums evolved without academic or clinical interdisciplinary collaboration. Training for new roles was built on the premise that physician support was paramount, and program philosophies were curative, competency levels of products variable, and their supervision questionable. Continuing career opportunities were not negotiated with existing professions. The medic-centered view emphasizing manpower shortages and the optimal numbers of personnel needed has misguided legislators, the public, and the health professionals themselves, preventing the formulation of creative, innovative, and viable national policies for health manpower development. New roles have been created without considering (or consulting with) presently existing groups. Options and alternatives to diversify within one's own professional or technical group was slowed by a host of impinging legal, traditional, and professional limitations. Sex discrimination, according to Cleland,[18] was another major deterrent to changes in roles.

Innovation in creating new manpower roles comes about, according to Robbins,[62] when the health care industry (or some enterprising health professional) can no longer tolerate the conservative "shortage mentality," defined by using only existing professional designations, in addressing manpower problems. New roles in nursing began to emerge during the 1960s.[8,11,21,35,36,45] Nursing gained recognition as an untapped source of readily available, trained manpower. Efforts by teams of nurses and physicians to prepare nurses to assume increasing responsibility for the delivery of health care began in the early 1960s. This concept, often labeled "nurse practitioner" or "nurse associate," was envisioned to improve the quality of health care, particularly health maintenance care. Expansion of the nurse's role included an increased competency in sophisticated assessment of the health status of individuals, managing health maintenance problems independently, working interdependently and collaboratively with physicians (and others) in curative functions, and, in essence, assuming a highly accountable professional role as a patient advocate, not a physician extender.

In the early '60s, experimentation in expanding the nurse's role in maternal and child care in ambulatory settings began. Ford and Silver,[34,35] and others[6,21] recorded their early efforts. With a colleague in the Medical School at the

University of Colorado, I developed the pediatric nurse practitioner project. This project was designed to prepare professional nurses at the post-baccalaureate level to provide comprehensive well-child care in ambulatory settings. This successful five-year demonstration project, the Primex projects,[46] and others similarly structured in universities and health agencies around the nation have served as trend setters, influencing both educational programs and health care delivery patterns. From the Colorado project and Lewis and Resnick's study[48] on the care of the chronically ill, nursing was catapulted into the limelight of health care. Because of reports on the success of these undertakings and other demonstrations and evaluations of the nurse's competency, consumer acceptance and the future potential of an expanded nurse's role are now a part of the record.

What has *not* been recognized, and is seldom written about, but which still holds great promise for future research in nursing practice, is the outcome in patient behavior following an experience with nurse practitioners. Nurse practitioners who use their new armamentarium and their commitment to accountability for helping the client become increasingly competent to care for himself and his family are a vital national resource. Little emphasis has been placed on the behavioral changes in consumers toward self-help or increasing potential that is offered through his learning experiences with a knowledgeable, accountable nurse practitioner. One major goal of this kind of clinical practice is to provide the consumer with feedback (data collected by interview and physical and psychosocial assessment) through conscious and directed strategies to help him become increasingly responsible for his own health. When the consumer actively participates, he can learn to explore options open to him and to make choices about his life style knowledgeably and wisely. These nurse practitioners are not physician extenders, but their role is complementary to the medical role. As patient/person/family advocate, the nurse practitioner meets needs in the prevention of illness and the promotion of health which are not adequately addressed in the current practice of any professional group. Research on the positive promotion of health is also needed.

Today, great doubt is expressed about the effectiveness, efficiency, and economy of multiple screening, annual physical examinations and other modalities employed to maintain optimal health. This doubt is a hopeful sign. Perhaps it will lead to extensive investigations to determine appropriate directions for a wiser utilization of the nation's resources. The tragedy is that all "health professionals" know much more about illness than health. Nursing must concern itself, for example, with certain daily living habits such as overeating, excessive alcohol intake, and smoking that are known to be detrimental to health. In essence, nurse practitioners can assume extensive accountability for groups of patients who have a myriad of unmet needs and who are incompetent in self-care and unskilled in their use of the health care system. People of all ages, including children, can become progressively more competent to care for themselves. They can learn to use the health care system aggressively and efficiently. They can influence community and national decisions about health care and make the system responsive to and responsible for changing needs and demands. In a democracy, people can foster the growth and development of a system that will help each individual live with his greatest potential for wellness. But people must value health. Further, they must be willing to establish priorities in allocating the necessary resources to attain health. Too little has been said about unmet health needs of populations, probably because most people don't really know—and will never learn from observing current health habits of professionals—that health is more than the absence of disease; that health can be viewed and valued as a means and mechanism for social change as well as an end in itself; that the joy of high level wellness contributes immeasurably to the happiness of individuals and influences greatly the worth and wealth of a nation. Regretfully, these lofty goals are seldom examined by consumers and providers who establish the traditional stereotyped relationships of other eras.

DeKock van Leeuwen[22] and Wise[81] present arguments concerning the basic relationship between health provider and consumer and the role of team delivery care that are worthy of consideration. They raise some basic questions about the reallocation of functions of highly trained people to lesser trained helpers. DeKock van Leeuwen postulates that the consumer seeks comfort from pain from *one* person, not a team, and that the physician provider needs some routine jobs between highly complex, puzzling patient visits to think about the patient's problems and the management of those problems. The professional worker cannot be bombarded constantly with intellectually taxing problems without occasional respites through visits with clients regarding simple and mundane problems. The underlying psychological dynamics of interpersonal relationships between patients and team members also come under scrutiny. Few health workers are prepared by their basic education programs to work together. Wise[81] substantiates this concern in the following comments by a consultant to the Martin Luther King, Jr. Health Center project:

> It is naive to bring together a highly diverse group of people and expect that, by calling them a team, they will in fact behave as a team. It is ironic indeed to realize that a football team spends 40 hours a week practicing teamwork for the two hours on Sunday afternoon when their team work really counts. Teams in organizations seldom spend two hours per year practicing when their ability to function as a team counts 40 hours per week [p. 444].

Concern for quality of care has replaced the numbers game in considering the problems of health care delivery. Flurries of activities to develop more sophisticated research and evaluative designs are apparent. Governmental influence, felt most sharply with the advent of the Professional Standards Review Program (P.S.R.O.) legislation,[43] is but a "sign of the times." Increasingly, state and federal governments are searching out ways to gain control of the health care industry. Regulatory agencies inaugurated to control costs, extend and improve delivery of care, and promote appropriate utilization of health care resources abound. In an astute analysis of creeping "regulationism," Inglehard[43] states:

This trend [toward stricter regulations] building the past two years, will accelerate dramatically in the near future. It began with regulation of prices charged by health institutions. But now it is being extended to the basic workings of the medical profession, to address the nature and quality of health services.

Great strides in meeting the health manpower needs of the nation cannot be made until a national policy for health and subsequently for health manpower is formulated. The present maldistribution of personnel, their fragmented and sporadic training, and their misutilization in antiquated health care delivery patterns combine to make the health care system (or nonsystem) episodic, chaotic, inefficient, and ineffective if measured by the goals of delivery of primary care and/or comprehensive care. A recent report from the Committee on Economic Development[20] declares that national policy for health could provide for "a drastic relocation of resources and an equally drastic reorganization of the health care delivery system."

Without the direction afforded by a national health manpower policy, we will be faced with increasing specialization, continuing maldistribution, and sporadic shortages and imbalances. The central strength of all health personnel may be dissipated and diverted once again into responses to crises rather than into innovative action for planned change. Regretfully, the deification of the physician as the central source of manpower makes thinking about old problems in new ways difficult. In the past, physicians, consumers, and some new health workers have conceived many new health manpower roles to be built on the delegation of tasks by physicians. The fallacy in this type of thinking is in the assumption that the health services as they now exist are excellent, if only the physician could be helped to do his job better. Recently, Magraw[51] refuted this assumption and suggested that interdependence in health care practice is evolving:

Most practitioners now in medicine have come to realize that independence in the present interdependent medical-care system is illusory and that it is incorrect to equate an avoidance of accommodation to that system with personal freedom. The maximizing of professional autonomy within the system is a more realistic style of work than insistence on a literal (and isolated) independence and self-sufficiency; participation in the system leaves greater time and energy for professional effectiveness and the pursuit of self-determined goals [p. 1407].

But changes in the health care system are paramount to altering the roles of health workers. The health care system today is a sick system, episodic and crisis-oriented. The system encourages and, indeed, demands that a person declare himself ill and requiring medical diagnosis rather than a health assessment and health maintenance plan. Rewards, in the form of attention and health insurance payments, are only given for identifiable diseases. Entry into the system for health maintenance is cumbersome and slow. If increased numbers of health workers (including nurses) are prepared to serve in the acute care system, the nation will continue the chaotic allocation of its financial and personnel resources to where 10 per cent of the population is found, namely, in hospitals. White[77] points out that, "The trick in the U.S. will be to encourage the evolution of health care arrangements and organizations that give reasonable choices to both consumers and physicians [and I add other health professionals], that provide responsible services and reasonable rates and that meet established standards for quality and equity of access" [p. 32].

In the past decade, neighborhood health centers have sought to meet the health needs and demands of deprived populations and a few health maintenance organizations and some innovative new patterns of delivering health care[2,14,66] have been inaugurated. Many of these efforts have included experimentation in the preparation and utilization of a variety of new categories of health personnel and/or redefining previous roles of workers. The efforts have generally demonstrated in a limited way that health care delivery can be different from the traditional systems of medical care. However, any permanent changes in the whole system will invariably require commitment to a philosophy of comprehensive health care, the deployment of personnel and financial resources to fulfill this commitment, and ways to measure the quality of care in terms of improvements in the health status of the populaion served.

Beyond a philosophical commitment, a framework for studying manpower problems will be necessary. One such framework, for the study of meeting health manpower needs in Colombia, was devised in 1963 by people from North and South America under grants from the Pan American Health Organization and the Milbank Memorial Fund. This framework, declared as vital to the development of national health manpower plans, is basic and pertinent to any future considerations in the United States. Its basic components are described by West[76]:

1. A profile of the health of the people, measured in terms of mortality, morbidity and other health indices—all related to demographic characteristics—age, sex, education, economic status and place of residence.

2. A picture of health services currently supplied—the effective demand—including physician visits, hospitalization and other services, again related to demographic data.

3. A picture of unmet health service needs and demands.

4. An inventory of present health manpower resources, estimates of functional productivity and projections of future supply.

5. A parellel picture of supply and utilization of hospitals and other health service facilities.

6. An appraisal of education resources available and the manpower pool on which they draw.

7. A study of education requirements for the future.

8. An assessment of the economic resources available for health services and education for such services.

9. Establishment of goals for health achievement related to present and projected resources and determination of the manpower requirements for those goals.

This approach to the formulation of national manpower policy and determination of manpower needs, deployment, utilization, and evaluation is in the best interest of the society that the health care system is designed to serve.

As this chapter goes to press, the *New York Times* reports that President Nixon has signed into law a "Bill for Reform in Medical Care."[57] The *Times* said that "the new law should help shift the emphasis of American Medical Care to the prevention of illness. A focus on prevention is widely considered more desirable, more efficient, and probably more economical than the present emphasis on treatment of illness that has already developed." The bill (Health Maintenance Act of 1973) provides for $375 million to establish and evaluate health maintenance organizations (HMOs) during the next five years. The HMO is described by Wilson[80] as:

. . . an organized system for delivering a broad spectrum of health services to an enrolled group of persons. The organization accepts a contractual responsibility for their care. It is a system designed to bring about health manpower, facilities, and consumers together into more effective relationships for meeting health care needs efficiently and in a manner convenient to the provider and consumer. It places emphasis upon preventive services [p. 7].

Emphasis on prevention is promoted by a reward system for maintaining wellness in subscribers and incentives for providers to use their skills and resources effectively, efficiently, and economically. The pluralistic, competitive nature of health care delivery is declared a strength by some political factions, but a weakness by others who believe health is too important to be a political issue. The fact of the matter is that health care is indeed a political issue—and a highly controversial one that no major politician can avoid addressing.

At the time the President signed the HMO bill, the nation was spending annually close to $80 billion or 7.6 per cent of the gross national product on health care. Proposals for new systems of health care through insurance programs had been introduced by both major political parties. The federal government's executive and congressional branches have joined together in a broad movement toward strict regulation of the health care industry.[43] State regulatory machinery to control institutional growth and costs for health care exists in nine states. Expanded Medicare and Medicaid legislation is predicted. Unionization of some health center and hospital staffs is bringing demands for increased wages and extensive benefits.

Changing legal statutes affecting the practice of both the old and the emerging categories of professional and technical health workers make analysis, preparation, distribution, and utilization of health manpower an even more complex, multifaceted problem. As new health workers arrived on the scene and new roles were generated, there was great agitation that resulted in changes in legislation governing practice and licensure of emerging categories of personnel. At one point in the late 1960s, a moratorium was called on expanding licensure to so many and such varied categories of personnel. Some states passed laws allowing the physician assistant to practice.[23,65] Changes in some state nurse practice acts, such as in Washington and New York, permitted expansion of the role of the nurse. At the end of the decade the concept of institutional licensure was introduced.[63] This concept, vehemently opposed by many nursing leaders, places the major responsibility for monitoring and controlling professional practice on institutions rather than the professional.

Concurrently, a struggle for the control of accreditation of programs preparing new health workers and certification for practice has emerged among the major professional association, i.e., the A.M.A., the A.N.A., and the A.A.P. Despite the early and heroic efforts to collaborate and coordinate activities of the National Joint Practice Committee (with some great personal sacrifices on the part of its member nurses and physicians), the relationships appear at this writing to have disintegrated. Territorial fights among providers have erupted. Nurses who have demonstrated courage and leadership in creating new roles for themselves will need to think carefully through the decisions regarding the source of accreditation and support for identifying credentials. If nurse practitioners are truly accountable to the society they serve and if their commitment is to *nursing* people, then it is difficult for me to believe that control of the professional practice of nursing will be given to any group outside the nursing profession. Indeed, medicine has not extended the prerogative of peer review, certification, or accreditation of its practitioners to any group other than itself.

No easy answers can or will be found. Implementation of the political and social goals of comprehensive health care for every American will require extensive exploration of feasibilities and the reordering of national priorities. Major changes in the organization, financing, and delivery of health care and in the preparation and practice of our 3.5 million health workers are essential future imperatives.

The current state of health manpower planning is outlined in a recent Washington News Letter of the American Public Health Association[7] as follows:

> New legislation that will severely curtail present levels of health manpower support will also be proposed. Institutional support on a formula basis is to be eliminated. A small amount of funds will be proposed for project grants for which all disciplines could compete.
> No extension of the existing authorities for public health training or allied health professions educational assistance is proposed.
> HEW predicts the possiblility of an oversupply of medical personnel if the training capacity continues to increase as it has in the past. The Department estimates that by 1985 we will have 50 percent more physicians, 40 percent more dentists and 80 percent more registered nurses than in 1970.

This news, coupled with the President's January 30, 1974, State of the Union message, has serious implications for consumers, providers, and educators. It points up the need for a national health policy to provide overall guidance for the preparation, financing, distribution, utilization, and evaluation of health manpower.

What's good for the provider *may* be good for the consumer and vice versa, but the prophetic statement of the President of General Motors has a hollow ring— witness the energy crisis.

To end these reflections on a more hopeful note, one has only to look at the new breed of professionals entering the health field. These bright, able young people whose sense of social responsibility and public concern will influence public policy, generate new models of interdisciplinary education and practice, involve the consumer creatively and energetically in decisions about health care, and raise eloquent and pertinent questions about the future of health care are our hope for the future. As Dr. Jonas Salk[67] says:

Answers pre-exist. It is the questions that need to be discovered.

REFERENCES

1. Adamson, T. E.: Critical issues in the use of physician associates and assistants. American Journal of Public Health 61:1765-1779, September 1971.
2. Abdellah, Faye G., et al.: New Directions in Patient-Centered Nursing. The MacMillan Company, New York, 1973.
3. American Medical Association: A Report on Education and Utilization of Allied Health Manpower. Chicago, June 1972.
4. American Medical Association: Allied Medical Education Newsletter, Vol. VI, No. 1, January 1, 1974.
5. American Medical Association: Expanding the Supply of Health Services in the 1970s. National Congress on Health Manpower, Chicago, October 22-24, 1970.
6. American Nurses Association and American Academy of Pediatrics: Child Health Care in the '70s. Report of Eastern Regional Workshop, New York, 1972.
7. American Public Health Association: Washington News Letter, No. 2, February 11, 1974, p. 3.
8. Andrews, Priscilla M., and Yankauer, Alfred: The pediatric nurse practitioner: Growth of the concept. American Journal of Nursing 71:504-506, March 1971.
9. Armiger, Sister Bernadette: Unemployment: Is there a nursing shortage? in Current Issues in Nursing Education. National League for Nursing, New York, 1973, pp. 26-30.
10. Barden, J. C.: Blue Cross will seek 8% rise in 1974 reimbursement rates. The New York Times, December 16, 1973.

11. Bates, Barbara: Doctor and nurse: Changing roles and relations. New England Journal of Medicine 283:129-134, July 1970.

12. Briney, K. L.: Manpower. Hospitals 45:121-130, April 1971.

13. Brook, Robert H.: Critical issues in the assessment of quality of care and their relationship to HMO's. Journal of Medical Education 48:114-134, April 1973.

14. Building a National Health Care System. Committee for Economic Development, 477 Madison Ave., New York, p. 80.

15. Bulletin of The New York Academy of Medicine, April, 1973.

16. Campbell, Rita R.: Economics of Health and Public Policy. American Enterprise Institute for Public Policy Research, Washington, 1971.

17. Chow, R. K.: Research + PRIMEX = improved health services. International Nursing Review 19:319-327, 1972, DHEW Publication No. (HSM) 73-3018.

18. Cleland, V.: Sex discrimination: Nursing's most pervasive problem. American Journal of Nursing 71:1542-1547, August 1971.

19. Colwill, Jack M.: The shifting emphasis in the delivery of health care—viewpoint of a physician, in Primary Health Care . . . Everybody's Business. National League for Nursing, New York, 1973, pp. 9-19.

20. Committee for Economic Development: Building a National Health-Care System. New York, 1973, p. 80.

21. Connelly, J. P., Stoeckle, J. D., Lepper, E. S., and Farrisey, R. M.: Physician and nurse—their interprofessional work in office and hospital ambulatory settings. New England Journal of Medicine 275:765-769, 1966.

22. DeKock van Leeuwen, J.A.C.: Some social and emotional aspects of health manpower planning. Medical Care 7:261-266, May-June 1969.

23. DMI Health Manpower Data, Physician Support Personnel. DHEW Publication No. (NIH) 72-183, Revised, May 1972.

24. Diers, Donna: It's a good time for nursing. Yale Alumni Magazine, December 1972, pp. 8-13.

25. Duff, R. S., Rowe, D. S., and Anderson, F. P.: Patient care and student learning in a pediatric clinic. Pediatrics 50:839-846, December 1972.

26. Ebert, Robert H.: Biomedical research policy—a re-evaluation. New England Journal of Medicine 289:348-375, August 1973.

27. Ebert, Robert H.: The medical school. Scientific American 229:138-142, September 1973.

28. Edwards, Charles C.: A candid look at health manpower problems. Journal of Medical Education 49:19-26, January 1974.

29. Egelston, E. M. and Kinser, T.: Licensure of hospital personnel—first of two articles. Hospitals 44:35-39, November 1970.

30. Extending the Scope of Nursing Practice. A Report of the Secretary's Committee to Study Extended Roles for Nurses, Department of Health, Education, and Welfare, November 1971.

31. Facts about Nursing 72-73. American Nurses Association, Kansas City, 1974, p. 14.
32. Ibid., p. 70.
33. Ibid., p. 98.
34. Feldstein, Martin S.: The medical economy. Scientific American 229:151-159, September 1973.
35. Ford, Loretta C., and Silver, Henry K.: The expanded role of the nurse in child care. Nursing Outlook 15:43-45, September 1967.
36. Ford, P. A., Seacat, M. S., and Silver, G. G.: Broadening roles of public health nurse and physician in prenatal and infant supervision. American Journal of Public Health 56:1097-1103, 1966.
37. Flook, E. Evelyn, and Sanazaro, Paul J., Editors: Health Services Research and R & D in Perspective. The University of Michigan, Health Administration Press, School of Public Health, Ann Arbor, 1973.
38. Fuchs, Victor R., and Kramer, Marcia J.: Determinants of Expenditures for Physicians' Services in the United States, 1948-68. Department of Health, Education, and Welfare, U. S. Government Printing Office, Washington, D.C., 1972.
39. Gerstein, Marc S., et al.: Factors Influencing the Expansion of the Nurse's Role in Primary Care Settings: A Study of the Graduates of a Nurse Practitioner Program. Massachusetts Institute of Technology, Cambridge, Massachusetts, 1973.
40. Green, M.: Naturalistic observations in a pediatric outpatient clinic. Pediatrics 50:849-852, December 1972.
41. Haggerty, R. J.: Patient care and student learning in a pediatric clinic. Pediatrics 50:847-848, December 1972.
42. Hughbanks, J. and Freeborn, D.: Review of twenty-two training programs for physician's assistants, 1969. HSMHA Health Reports 86:857-862, October 1971.
43. Igelhart, J. K.: Health report/Executive-congressional coalition seeks tighter regulation for medical-services industry. National Journal Reports, November 10, 1973, pp. 1684-1692.
44. Josiah Macy, Jr. Foundation: The Greater Medical Profession. Report of a Symposium of The Royal Society of Medicine and the Josiah Macy, Jr. Foundation, New York, 1973.
45. Kendall, Katherine: Sixteenth International Confederation of Midwives Congress. MCH Exchange 2:8, December 1972.
46. Leininger, Madeleine, Little, D. E., and Carnevali, Doris: Primex. American Journal of Nursing 72:1274-1277, July 1972.
47. Lewis, Charles E., and Resnick, Barbara A.: Nurse clinics and progressive ambulatory patient care. New England Journal of Medicine 277:1236-1241, December 1967.
48. Lewis, Charles E., Resnick, Barbara A., Schmidt, Glenda, and Waxman,

          David: Activities, events, and outcomes in ambulatory patient care. New
          England Journal of Medicine 280:645-649, March 1969.
49.   Little, Dolores E.: Health providers—new patterns: Role of the nurse, in
      Hospital Care in the '70's . . . Forces for Change. National League for
      Nursing, New York, 1973, pp. 18-21.
50.   Losee, Garrie J., and Altenderfer, Marion E.: Health Manpower in Hos-
      pitals. U. S. Government Printing Office, Washington, D.C., 1970.
51.   Magraw, R. M.: Trends in medical education and health services—their im-
      plications for a career in family medicine. New England Journal of
      Medicine 285:1407-1413, December 1971.
52.   Molloy, Gail: Pediatric nurse practitioner program. Journal of the New York
      State Nurses Association 4:21-23, September 1973.
53.   Miller, J. D., and Ferber, B.: Health manpower in the 1960s. Hospitals
      45:66-71, February 1971.
54.   National Commission for the Study of Nursing and Nursing Education, Je-
      rome P. Lysaught, Director: An Abstract for Action. McGraw Hill Book
      Co., New York, 1970.
55.   National Health Council, Inc.: The Changing Role of the Public and Private
      Sectors in Health Care. Chicago, 1973.
56.   National League for Nursing: Current Issues in Nursing Education. New
      York, 1972.
57.   New York Times, December 30, 1973, p. 1.
58.   Nurse Supply and Needs: Current Nursing Statistics in Brief. DHEW
      Publication No. (HRA) 74-18, Revised, 1973.
59.   Nurses, in the Extended Role, are not Physicians' Assistants. American
      Nurse's Association, Inc., mimeographed letter, July 9, 1973.
60.   Pennell, Maryland Y., and Hoover, David B.: Health Manpower Source
      Book, Section 21, Allied Health Manpower Supply and Requirements.
      U. S. Government Printing Office, Washington, D.C., 1970, pp. 1950-
      1980.
61.   Physician's Assistant Examination, in Chronicle of Higher Education, Vol.
      VIII, No. 3, October 9, 1973.
62.   Robbins, Anthony: Allied health manpower. The New England Journal of
      Medicine 286:918-923, April 1972.
63.   Roemer, Ruth: Legal regulation of modern nursing practice, in Current
      Issues in Nursing Education. National League for Nursing, New York,
      1973, pp. 15-25.
64.   Rogers, M. E.: Eulogy to Obsolescence: A.N.A. Board Statement on
      "Graduates of Diploma Schools of Nursing." Mimeograph distribution,
      1973.
65.   Sadler, A. M., Jr., Sadler, Blair L., and Bliss, Ann A.: The Physician's
      Assistant—Today and Tomorrow. Yale University School of Medicine,
      1972, pp. 253.

66. Saward, Ernest W.: The organization of medical care. Scientific American 229:169-175, September 1973.
67. Salk, Jonas: The National Foundation/March of Dimes Annual Report, 1973, p. 22.
68. Schlotfeldt, R. M.: This I believe . . . Nursing is health care. Nursing Outlook 20:245-246, April 1972.
69. Schwartz, W. B.: Policy Analysis and the Institute of Medicine. Paper delivered to Spring Meeting, Institute of Medicine, National Academy of Sciences, Washington, May 10, 1972.
70. Siegel, Earl, and Bryson, Sylvia L.: Redefinition of the role of the public health nurse in child health supervision. American Journal of Public Health 53:1015-1024, July 1963.
71. Stanton, Marjorie: The baccalaureate program. Journal of the New York State Nurses Association 4:16-19, September 1973.
72. Storms, Doris M.: Training of the Nurse Practitioner: A Clinical and Statistical Analysis. Connecticut Health Services Research Series No. 4, North Haven, Connecticut, 1973.
73. U. S. Department of Health, Education, and Welfare: Selected Training Programs for Physician Support Personnel. U. S. Government Printing Office, Washington, D.C., Rev. 1972.
74. U. S. Department of Health, Education, and Welfare: The Size and Shape of the Medical Care Dollar. U. S. Government Printing Office, Washington, D.C., 1972.
75. U. S. Department of Health, Education, and Welfare: Technology and Health Care in the 1980's. U. S. Government Printing Office, Washington, D.C., 1972.
76. West, Margaret D.: Colombian National Health Survey: Planning, Methods, Operation, in Research Methods in Health Care, PRODIST John B. McKinlay, ed. New York, 1973, pp. 135-136.
77. White, Kerr L.: Life and death and medicine. Scientific American 229:22-33, September 1973.
78. Whittington, H. G.: The Mental Health Practitioner. Hospitals 44:52-54, November 1970.
79. Wilber, J. A., and Barrow, J. G.: Hypertension—a community problem. American Journal of Medicine 52:653-663, May 1972.
80. Wilson, Vernon E.: HMO's: Hopes and aspirations. Journal of Medical Education 48:7-10, April 1973.
81. Wise, Harold: The primary care health team. Archives of International Medicine 130:444, September 1972.
82. Young, Robert L.: Apples and oranges and bananas—diversity in a health manpower consortium. American Journal of Public Health 64:140-143, February 1974.

Health Care Trends
and Nursing Roles*

JOHN H. BRYANT, M.D.

INTRODUCTION

The health care system is in a period of marked change, and those changes will affect virtually all health professionals—their roles, their interrelations with one another, and their educational preparation.

Despite the obvious need for change in the health care system and the eagerness of those who work within the system to reduce barriers to quality care and facilitate change, the complexity, ponderousness, and inherent inertia of the system mitigate against rapid or radical change. This is an example of what Schon[7] calls dynamic conservatism, or the tendency of persons, institutions, and systems to keep things the same. Our own health care system is particularly likely to exhibit these characteristics because of its pluralism, expressed in this instance by the dispersion of power centers and the lack of organizational arrangements that might bring those power centers together in common action for change. Thus, the inertia is great and the forces of change, while substantial in number, are not concerted in direction.

While this time of change will affect all health professions, it will be particularly challenging for nursing. There are three reasons for this: First, there has been a turbulence within nursing and between nursing and medicine concerning the mission of nursing and how to translate that mission into nursing roles and nursing education. At a time when our society awaits a response as to how many of its unmet needs nursing can meet, nursing is trying to determine its historical problem of mission and professional identity.

Second, there is a major health manpower gap in the provision of primary care. It is logical for nursing to fill that gap, but there are differing views as to what this opportunity represents or what the response of nursing should be. Nursing's moves toward filling the gap will be made difficult not only by the intricacies of

---

*Adapted from a presentation to the Conference on Distributive Nursing, Duke University School of Nursing.

roles and role interrelationships, but also by the sheer numbers of persons involved, which can mean nearly tidal shifts in nursing education and placement.

Third, nursing needs to bring a substantial research effort to bear on the implications for nursing of changes in the health care system. The future shape of the system is unclear and the roles that seem to be beckoning to nursing are not well defined. The fluidity and importance of these require that new initiatives be built on the solid ground of careful observation and experimentation.

Overall, the evolution of the health care system is crucial for nursing. Nursing and other health professions must be responsive to evolving patterns of care, the increasing need for primary care providers being an example. Recent history indicates that if nursing does not respond to the needs of the system, others will. An example is the emergence of the physician's assistant while nursing was either rejecting the concept or moving very slowly toward extending the clinical functions of nurses.

At the same time, the decisions made by nursing will be crucial for the health care system. Nursing represents an extraordinary manpower resource in terms of both number and quality, with potential for adaptation to a wide variety of health care functions. The trends that emerge in nursing are bound to influence the shape and function of the system. Two examples are the emergence of nurse practitioners and the revisions of the nurse practice law in many states that make it lawful for nurses to practice independently, without the supervision of physicians.

It is this interrelationship between trends in health care and the current as well as potential roles of nursing to which we should be alert.

THE EVOLVING HEALTH CARE SYSTEM

The pluralism and complexity of the health system make it exceedingly difficult to undertake a wholistic analysis of the major problems in health care and their relationships to one another. Accordingly, this chapter will be a listing and brief discussion of 10 components of the system, followed by reflections on what has been referred to as "distributive nursing."

Changing Patterns of Ambulatory Care

The Network Problem. The major trouble spot in the health care system is ambulatory care, and the troubles are felt most seriously in rural and inner city areas. Most of the troubles can be grouped under what might be called the network problem.

Providers of health care frequently function in isolation from one another, even though they may be located in the same geographical area. This isolation applies not only to hospitals, group practices, and municipal health stations, but also to physicians, many of whom have no effective relationships with hospitals. The lack of an adequate network results in duplication of some services, omission of others, and overall, an uneven distribution of services.

Patients are often limited in their access to physicians and unclear about how to gain access to any health care at all. They may either fail to obtain care or, at the other extreme, make an unnecessary number of visits to providers.

The movement of patients between providers is often not associated with useful exchanges of medical information. Lacking both medical information and a continuity of relationship with patients, physicians and nurses often have little choice but to take an episodic, disease-oriented approach instead of one that focuses on the total health needs of patients. Since continuity of care is dependent to some extent on health personnel having information that describes the full range of a patient's problems and care, changes might be required that will put relevant information into the hands of nurses or physicians whose roles are to provide only part of a patient's care.

At the center of these network problems is the public's increasing use of hospital emergency departments. Since emergency rooms are often the front doors of hospitals, patients enter them in large numbers on an unscheduled basis with a wide range of problems, from simple to complex. These facilities, designed and staffed to handle true emergencies in relatively small numbers, have great difficulty in adapting to the sheer weight of numbers and variety of demand. These events are forcing changes in the outlook and functions of hospital administrators, physicians, nurses, and educators, as they recognize that entirely new or revised concepts are involved in the management of patient flow, disposition decisions, health team compositions, interpersonal relationships between clinic personnel and patients, methods of paying for services, and so forth.

Another problem in ambulatory care is inadequate arrangement for areawide planning and coordination. Events within the ambulatory care sector of the hospital are usually not effectively related to events outside the hospital. The ways providers relate to one another and to their communities fail to facilitate efficient delivery of health services, much less areawide planning. There is no local health authority in New York City, for example, with overall responsibility for health care. The Department of Health, which has statutory authority to "promote the public health," concentrates its resources chiefly on specific preventive programs and, increasingly, on monitoring and evaluating health care programs. The Comprehensive Health Planning Agency, which is intended to coordinate health services in the city and assure consumer participation and management, still lacks a plan and the statutory authority to enforce it. Thus, while the totality of health care resources is considerable, actually reducing barriers to care and facilitating access, effectiveness, and efficiency of care will require substantial innovations. Such innovations are being introduced on at least three fronts, and the participation of nursing is essential in each instance.

First is the development of more effective relationships among the various providers so as to facilitate patient access to primary care, to provide better referral of patients for secondary and tertiary care, and to ensure prompt transfer of appropriate medical information among providers. The isolated pieces need to be brought together into a functioning network.

Second is the improvement of ambulatory care units of the major hospitals, most of which require better management of unscheduled visits and more effective linkages with other providers of health services, particularly with respect to referral and consultative relationships. The hospitals need to be strengthened so they can more effectively support the network.

The third front is the development of areawide health services research, planning, and evaluation capability. The network needs to make unified decisions and show that it can be responsive to the demands and needs of specific population constituencies, such as children, the elderly, and so forth, in a given geographical area. The research component should be practically oriented toward health problems and health care needs. Planning should include providers, consumers, governmental agencies, and fiscal intermediaries and should be directed toward making the best use of resources, including health manpower, in providing health care for defined populations. Evaluation should be oriented toward measures of health status and/or health care needs and means for monitoring the quality and cost of care. It remains to be seen to what extent recently enacted and projected legislation regarding areawide planning, health services research, and professional services review organizations will facilitate the development of effective areawide planning and coordinating.

Community Hospitals. Community hospitals will play an increasingly important role in ambulatory care in the coming years. In 1972, there were more than 200 million visits to hospitals in the United States, three-quarters of these to community hospital clinics and emergency rooms. In comparison, there were less than 20 million visits to prepaid group practices and neighborhood health centers. Of the 6,000 community hospitals in the United States, only 15 per cent are affiliated with medical schools or accredited as teaching hospitals. Thus, 85 per cent of all outpatient hospital visits are outside the orbit of academic health services. Community hospitals can capitalize on their unique ability to mobilize resources and attract, organize, and deploy the physicians, nurses, and allied workers who have the training and skills to maintain health, treat illness, and contribute to reform in ambulatory care.[4] There is certain to be an expansion of the roles of hospitals beyond the provision of acute care to include more extensive ambulatory care, skilled nursing or long-term care, home health care, satellite clinics, telephone consultation systems, and a variety of experiments in collaborative relationships with other providers including hospital-related group practice.

Here, then, in the setting of community hospitals and their surrounding communities across the nation, is a trend of potentially great significance for nursing, particularly as nursing might contribute to the development of soundly conceived approaches to health care and maintenance.

New Arrangements for Financing Health Care

National health insurance is the focus of the most important debate on health care of this decade, and while the details are not yet clear it is highly probable that national health insurance legislation will become a reality in 1975 or 1976, thus reducing financial barriers to health care for a substantial part of the population.

The trend toward more prepaid health care programs, many of them with a fee-for-service component, will be accelerated by the Health Maintenance Organization concept and by the incorporation of provisions for more comprehensive and largely prepaid health care plans into labor-management negotiations. These changing patterns of payment for health care will affect all levels of the system, including nursing. For example, the evolution of nursing functions will be strongly influenced by policies on which functions will be paid through health insurance mechanisms.

Increasing Concern for Providing Health Care for Defined Populations

Health care in the United States traditionally has been oriented toward individuals who seek care. There is an increasing recognition, however, that many in need of health care do not seek it because they do not know they need it, do not know how to seek it, or are afraid to seek it. The elderly, for example, often live alone and are indigent, demoralized, and frightened; their plea for health care often comes late in the course of an illness that is by then destructive and expensive.

Providing care for those in need whether or not they seek care will be a substantial change, but it will come, and it will have important and radical implications for nursing, as discussed below.

Evaluation and Monitoring of the Quality and Cost of Health Care

There is widespread concern about our limitations in evaluating and monitoring the quality and cost of health care. Such evaluation is important not only for improving the quality and constraining the costs of care, but also as a mechanism for feeding back judgements on personnel performance and education and utilization of health manpower.

The main mechanism for evaluation and monitoring that is now on the legislative books is the Professional Services Review Organization program. Implementation of that program is moving very rapidly, but it remains to be seen how effective it is. Whether or not it is effective, perhaps the main thing to be said for the future is that evaluation and monitoring will be increasingly integral to the health care effort, and nursing should be closely involved with it. The attempt of the nursing profession to broaden the concept of "professional" in PSROs to include nurses as well as physicians is an example of this point.

Increasing Trend Toward Patient and Community Education

Patient and community education is increasingly being reorganized as an essential component of health care. This need is most simply illustrated by the large number of mothers who bring their children for the kind of health care that can be handled at home by better instructed mothers. Three major points can be made concerning this complicated field.

First, we need to be careful about equating education with mass media. While appreciating that some education can be achieved through television and the printed word, many problems within the scope of patient and community education may not be touched by this mode. Teaching mothers to cope with daily stresses, for example, may best be handled in a group with other mothers in the language and style of their own lives.

Second, providers of health care are often so firmly oriented toward patients seeking care for sickness that they fail to recognize other reasons for coming. The overt complaint may be masking a cry for help for an unmentioned and often nonmedical problem. Nurses can be particularly sensitive to this "help seeking" behavior.

Third, the health professions have not been notably successful in identifying those issues that patients and communities feel are most important in their education. Patients and communities should participate in developing educational programs directed toward their needs.

It is possible that the costs of health education will soon be reimbursable under federally financed health services, which would encourage giving increased emphasis to this important area.

Community Participation in Health Care Decisions

The trend toward community participation in the governance of health care programs and facilities appears to have moved from the earlier phases of disruptive confrontation (that was often necessary for communities to gain seats at decision-making tables) to a search for more constructive arrangements through which consumers and providers can build a mutual understanding on which to base health care decisions. Confrontation is still with us, however, and needs to be recognized as a normal ingredient of relationships among power centers in our pluralistic system. The challenge is to learn to work effectively in these confrontation relationships and to recognize the positive outcomes that are possible when the substantial resources of communities are enlisted in the health care enterprise.

New Relationships Between Academic Health Centers and the Health Care System

It is no longer rationally acceptable to isolate educational programs for different health personnel nor to plan those programs without an intimate and ongoing research-based understanding of the dynamics and manpower needs of changing health care arrangements. The now glaring irrelevancies in our educational programs to the needs of our evolving health care system, the tensions in relationships among health personnel, the need to bring research methods to bear on the forms and functions of health teams and on the educational programs to prepare students for health teams are all forces driving educational institutions to find more effective ways of structuring themselves. This structuring must have an internal focus with respect to the interrelationships among health professional schools, and an external focus with respect to health care delivery systems.

The variety of sizes, shapes, and compositions of health teams is mind-boggling. While one problem is to develop a rational basis for matching health teams to health care needs, another is to integrate educational programs with one another so that students will be educated for working within teams. In this connection, a task force of the Institute of Medicine of the National Academy of Sciences[6] studying the problem of interdisciplinary teaching made the following recommendations:

Every academic health center (an academic health center comprises two or more health professional schools, usually in association with multiple health care settings) has an obligation to engage in interdisciplinary education and extend its responsibility for fostering optimal cooperation among health professionals in the delivery of care.

Areawide planning of health care and the education of health personnel is having increasing practical manifestations. In recent years, regional planning bodies under Hill-Burton legislation, Regional Medical Programs, and Comprehensive Health Planning, have had limited success, partly because they were the product of political compromise and national inexperience. Nonetheless, it is virtually certain that there will be increasing rather than lessening efforts to develop effective areawide planning machinery. Legislation that is now being formulated contains such provisions. An ingredient that may not appear immediately in legislation (but probably will in the near future) is areawide planning of educational programs for health personnel to encourage cooperation among institutions, reduce duplication, maximize the use of limited educational resources, promote interdisciplinary education, and develop more effective connections between educational and health care programs.

Nursing has contributed to and needs to continue to participate in the development of different approaches to these complex problems.

Increased Concern for Health Manpower Planning

Health manpower planning, one of the weakest parts of our system,[2] has three identifiable components: monitoring supply, defining requirements, and influencing or controlling production and distribution. We will look briefly at each.

The data base and administrative arrangements for monitoring the supply of health manpower are limited in quality and effectiveness. The data are fairly accurate for physicians and dentists, of modest quality for nurses, and of poor quality for allied health personnel.

The art of defining health manpower requirements for our changing health care system borders on the primitive. Gaining agreement as to what constitutes desirable numbers and types of health personnel in differing settings is difficult even among those best informed. The complexities of determining system requirements for health manpower simply exceed our current capability for dealing with them.

We can identify examples of serious maldistributions of health personnel by specialty and by location, but there are currently few mechanisms for seriously influencing or controlling those imbalances. A number of professional associations, governmental agencies, and congressional committees are examining the problem and exploring possible solutions.

Thus, there will be increasing efforts to monitor the supply, more precisely define requirements, and develop modes for influencing or even controlling the production and distribution of health manpower. Rational nationwide or areawide planning of the education and utilization of nursing personnel should be at the forefront of the concerns of nursing.

Increasing Technological Developments

A listing of future trends would be incomplete without acknowledging the continued rapid development of the technological aspects of biomedical science including advances in bioengineering, radiological and sonic detection systems, sophisticated patient monitoring systems, surgical techniques, data storing processing and computing systems, new forms of maintaining and using patient records, the uses of an increasing variety of therapeutic drugs, and so forth. This short list of wide-spread advances tells us something about the rate of change in our health care capabilities and about the knowledge base required to participate effectively as health care practitioners.

Increasing Concern for Ethical and Moral Issues

An important companion to increasing technological developments, often seen as potentially dehumanizing, is a countertrend of increasing concern for the value of human life, the importance of individuality, the right to privacy, the dignity that should be associated with suffering and dying, the moral and social pitfalls in some forms of health care and human experimentation, and the problems of equitable distribution of health care. All of these reflect a healthy societal concern for human values.

IMPLICATIONS OF HEALTH CARE TRENDS FOR NURSING

A number of issues emerge from this review of health care trends that are important to nursing. Of particular importance are the ways in which nursing functions are evolving throughout the range of health care settings including hospitals and other health facilities, communities, and homes. The National Commission for the Study of Nursing and Nursing Education addressed this subject in detail and defined two career patterns:[3]

a) One career pattern, *episodic,* would emphasize the nursing practice that is essentially curative and restorative, generally acute or chronic in nature, and most frequently provided in the setting of a hospital or inpatient facility.

b) The second career pattern, *distributive,* would emphasize the nursing practice that is essentially designed for health maintenance and disease pre-

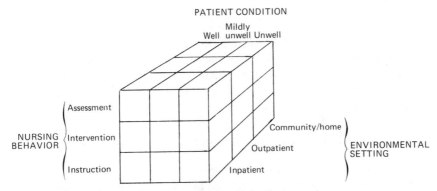

FIGURE 1. Interacting variables involved in episodic and distributive nursing.

vention. This is generally continuous in nature, seldom acute, and increasingly would take place in community or emerging institutional settings.

These concepts are represented by a three dimensional model with three interacting variables—nursing behavior (assessment, intervention, instruction), patient condition (well, mildly unwell, unwell), and environmental setting (inpatient center, outpatient facility, community and home) (see Fig. 1).

Two issues relating to distributive and episodic nursing will be considered, one having to do with their interrelationships, the other with the relationships between distributive nursing and distributive justice.

Distributive and Episodic Nursing—A False Dichotomy

The Commission Report[3] contrasts and separates episodic and distributive nursing. Episodic nursing has to do with curing or caring for patients with acute or chronic health problems in an inpatient setting; distributive nursing has to do with health maintenance and disease prevention, seldom with acute care, and generally takes place outside the hospital. While the Commission describes the interaction of the two and handles their interrelationships in a well balanced way (and states that there should be no chasm between the two), there is room to fear that the separation will stick in the minds of others and find its way into educational and career programs.

A twofold criticism of the potential separation of episodic and distributive functions is worth considering. First, the separation of functions is unlikely to be effective in the health care system. It has been tried in many places, the formerly French area of West Africa and New York City, for example, and it has not worked well, which is why the Child Health Stations in New York City are being converted from well child care to well *and* sick child care centers. A corollary of that change is that nurses who work in those converted stations will handle both well and sick children. If sick people cannot get primary care from the persons who are responsible for health maintenance functions, then the main possibility for continuity of care is intercepted.

A second criticism of the dichotomy has to do with the other side of the coin—the fact that the time of sickness is also a time when some of the most important steps toward the prevention of disease or further complications and the maintenance of health can take place. Thus prevention and treatment come together again.

The concepts of distributive and episodic nursing are useful, but it would be clearer conceptually if distributive nursing described the entire spectrum of care, with episodic nursing as one part of it.

Distributive Care and Health Care for Populations

The interactive model and the language describing it have to do with the care of *individual patients* in a variety of settings. Let me suggest that this concept is too narrow and that distributive nursing should include the care of populations, despite the facts that some aspects of the population care takes nurses away from individual patient care and that the ethical and technical issues involved may be new to many nursing curricula.

I suggest that *distributive nursing* be interpreted to mean that nursing care should be distributed according to the life needs of patients, their families, and communities. (Episodic care is considered to be a part of distributive care.) The fact that resources are not adequate to meet all those needs brings this concept of *distributive nursing* together with that of *distributive justice*. Let us consider some relationships between justice and health care.

Perhaps the most important modern thinker on the question of justice in the Western tradition is John Rawls of Harvard University. His influencial book, *A Theory of Justice*,[5] opens with the following statements:

Justice is the first virtue of social institutions, as truth is of systems of thought. A theory however elegant and economical must be rejected or revised if it is untrue; likewise laws and institutions no matter how efficient and well-arranged must be reformed or abolished if they are unjust. Each person possesses an inviolability founded on justice that even the welfare of society as a whole cannot override. For this reason justice denies that the loss of freedom for some is made right by a greater good shared by others. Therefore in a just society, the liberties of equal citizenship are taken as settled; the rights secured by justice are not subject to political bargaining or the calculus of social interest.

Rawls develops two principles of justice, one having to do with political and civil liberties, the other with the distribution of social and economic goods and burdens. The two are combined in a general conception of justice: that all social primary goods are to be distributed equally unless an unequal distribution of any or all of these goods is to the advantage of the least favored. Rawls' principle of justice in relation to health care can be expressed as follows:[1]

Whatever health care is available should be equally available to all. Departures from that equality of distribution are permissible only if those worse off are made better off.

Obviously there are great discrepancies between this principle and the way health care is provided in most countries. What guidelines can be offered for the development of health services that are more just?

Some secondary principles of justice related to health care are helpful, such as: *There should be a floor or minimum of health services for all.* Exceptions to this would be conditions of dire insufficiency where a floor would be meaningless. A floor of service should not be construed as an optimum but as the least that can be made available to all or nearly all. *Resources above the floor should be distributed according to need.* One of the most difficult questions to be faced in health care has to do with how to decide whom to serve when resources are inadequate to serve all. The question is usually ignored and care is provided for some, such as those who seek it, while others receive little or no care, even though they may be in serious need of it.

Justice would be met by using some of the health care resources for those in greatest need. To do so, however, requires first taking the needs of the entire population into account and then deciding who is in greatest need. Speaking theoretically and from the individual's point of view, justice is done when one's needs are taken into account, even though one's needs might not be met. Injustice lies not in not receiving care, but in not having one's needs taken into account in decisions about who should receive care.

The principle is made operationally practical by assessing the needs of defined populations, setting priorities in terms of health problems and population groups, developing programs for the best use of resources in caring for those problems and population groups, and, in the course of doing so, reaching those individuals in greatest need. For example, a survey of a population or local experience may reveal that health problems of the elderly and complications of pregnancy and childbirth are major problems. These may be given priority, but resources might be inadequate to provide care for all of the elderly and all pregnant women. A simple screening system can search through the population, identifying the elderly most in need and the women most at risk to develop complications during pregnancy and childbirth. These people can then be cared for to the extent that resources are available.

Thus, a just distribution of nursing (distributive nursing?) and other forms of health care would involve concern for all the people within a population, for those who seek care and those who do not. To broaden the concern of nursing in this way requires, first, that the nurse is part of a team and of a health care system with the capability for approaching the population much as the patient is approached (see Fig. 1): the needs of the population and of individuals are *assessed;* health care workers *intervene,* providing a floor of services for all, seeking out those most in need, and providing care or monitoring the process whereby they receive care. *Instruction* or education may be an important component of care.

To the extent that this process is not followed and the population is in need and not seeking care, or seeking and not receiving the care they need, then individuals in need will be lost from sight and suffer unnecessarily. By virtue of its historical commitment to the needs of individuals and its role of providing care or facilitating the process whereby care is provided, nursing is well suited to this extended concept of distributive nursing. This function may be seen as taking nursing further away from a concern for individual patients. The paradox is, however, that only a concern for all—a statistical concern—can insure that individuals receive the care they need.

REFERENCES

1. Bryant, John: Principles of Distributive Justice as a Basis for Designing a Health Care System. (Submitted for publication, 1974.)

2. Bryant, John: Health manpower planning in the changing scene of the 1970's. Mount Sinai Journal of Medicine, 40:576, 1973.

3. Lysaught, Jerome: An Abstract for Action; A report of the National Commission for the Study of Nursing and Nursing Education. McGraw-Hill Book Company, New York, 1970.

4. Olendski, M.O., Piore, N., Goldsmith, S.B., Ginsberg, A.G., and Bryant, J.H.: Community Hospital Related Group Practice. (In preparation, 1974.)

5. Rawls, John: A Theory of Justice. Harvard University Press, Cambridge, Mass., 1971.

6. Conference on Interrelationships of Educational Programs for Health Personnel, Institute of Medicine, Washington, D.C., April 1973.

7. Schon, Donald: Beyond the Stable State. Random House, New York, 1971.

The Quality of General Medical Services by Dentists*

PETER MILGROM, D.D.S.[†]

Hidden from view and rarely appreciated by patients are important general medical services furnished by dentists. Responsibility for the medical sequelae of dental treatment and the detection and followup of the oral and perioral signs of systemic disease are crucial concerns for dental practice. The dentist is a primary care practitioner. He should serve as a preventive health counselor and facilitator of good quality medical care.

This chapter contrasts the changing role of the dentist with the traditional model of practice, discusses the importance of this trend, and delineates specific areas of medical responsibility for the dentist. A major purpose will be to examine a dysfunction in patient care that has occurred in the dental profession and the efforts of dentists to incorporate the general medical sciences into their everyday practice. In our research, my associates and I have looked at specific adverse and quite clearly avoidable outcomes from dental treatment and have observed a discontinuity of educational opportunities for practicing dentists.[14] The central conclusion of this chapter is that a major effort to re-educate dentists to markedly broaden their knowledge of the general medical sciences is needed. Dental clinician-educators are a key target population for such a program. Boards of dental examiners must be charged by their state legislatures with identifying adverse and avoidable outcomes resulting from obsolescent standards of practice. Incentives should be developed for change.

Dental disease is common. A national survey[3] conducted between 1960 and 1962 found that the average American had at least 20 to 32 teeth missing, filled, or

---

*This report is a part of an ongoing research project, "Quality Control of End-Results: Identifying Avoidable Adverse Events in Dentistry," by the author. The participation of Drs. John I. Ingle, Hubert A. McGuirl, Burton Pollack, and Laurence R. Tancredi is gratefully acknowledged.

†Supported under a fellowship award from the Commonwealth Fund while Professional Associate, Institute of Medicine, National Academy of Sciences, Washington, D.C.

decayed and that three of four adults with natural teeth showed evidence of chronic periodontal infection. Interviews by the National Opinion Research Center have shown that the knowledge people have of how to care for their teeth exceeds their level of interest in obtaining treatment.[7,18] In this country, there is an estimated backlog of over 800 million unfilled cavities caused by tooth decay alone. During 1971, 59 per cent of the population visited the dentist at least once.[4] However, 10 per cent of the population utilized over 60 per cent of all dental appointments, and most of these visits were for symptomatic relief.[10] In general, it is unlikely that the public is very knowledgeable about the medical component of complete oral care.

It is evident, however, that many consumers are concerned about the problems of obtaining high quality health care.[17] Surveys[23] have reported a concern regarding unnecessary red tape associated with health insurance. Nonetheless, significant new groups of consumers are beginning to win contract benefits for dental care.[3] With increased utilization of services, the public is likely to become increasingly knowledgeable and discerning regarding the quality of services they receive. Public advocates, such as H. S. Denenberg, formerly of the Pennsylvania Department of Insurance, are making efforts to help consumers learn about dental care. Denenberg's *Shopper's Guide to Dentistry*,[5] for example, gives explicit requirements for the information a patient should get from a dentist before consenting to treatment. Alternative treatments, possible complications, and procedures are included. Denenberg suggests that no patient should patronize a dentist who is afraid of using consultation. Presently, few dentists obtain consultations, but as dental patients approach the dentist with more questions and requests for information, the dentist must be prepared to meet these requests in order to render high quality services.

Traditionally, the scope of dental practice has been limited, partially because the primary modes of dental surgery are relatively primitive. There has been an emphasis on symptomatic treatment for the relief of pain. Dentists have historically treated only well patients in their private offices, often neglecting chronically ill, aged, and institutionalized patients. Emphasis has also been on the quality of the single restoration or filling, rather than on the entire oral cavity, the head and neck, and the client's general health or total concerns. Standards for practice have been traditional in orientation, and largely reflect routine empirical clinical practices. Traditional dental practice is typified in a report by Friedman[6] regarding what he calls "mutilation by consensus." He reports that the single dental service provided to the majority of elderly patients is extraction of their teeth and states unequivocally that dentists have contributed to this situation. Frequently, elderly patients are not told of alternative treatments that may save their remaining teeth. Moreover, pricing schedules create economic incentives for extractions. This trend is a carry-over from when dental care provided fewer options than are possible today.

RECENT TRENDS AND NEW RESPONSIBILITIES

Dentistry is in a state of flux. One index for broadening dental services has been the growth of specialization. In recent years, the remarkable rise in the number of dentists electing specialty training has resulted, in part, in a partitioning of responsibility and in dentists finding difficulty in maintaining competence in the several treatment areas. There have been tremendous improvements in the instrumentation used in dental surgery. The high speed drill, for example, has vastly simplified technical procedures, and, consequently, dental auxilaries are being prepared to assume some routine aspects of restorative care. Important strides have been made in improving the capability for control of pain and anxiety in dental practice. This capability needs to be incorporated into everyday practice. An important trend in dental schools has been the increased emphasis on the detection and followup of systemic disease processes. In the last decade, there has been impressive growth in the areas of oral biology and community-based dentistry. Today, dentists are more skilled in medical services than in the past. Since the advent of Medicare, more elderly patients have had the resources to consult the dentist. An indication of increased demand for denture prosthesis is markedly higher cost.[13] The increasing use of drugs in medical therapy means that more dental patients have access to medications which may affect dental practices; thus the dentist must be more aware of these aspects of general medical care. Changing consumer demands and health practices are helping to broaden the definition of dentistry today.

Some new areas of responsibility for the dentist can be delineated by looking at dental care in relation to diagnosis, treatment, and followup. In the diagnostic process, a dentist is now expected to obtain a patient history that includes medical and social questions.[21] Today, the dentist is more aware of the reasons for asking specific health questions and is more apt, for example, to follow up on suspicious patient responses to a check-list type of questionnaire. The oral examination will include more than the teeth, as a good diagnostic evaluation includes an inspection of the soft tissues of the mouth and palpation of the glands and muscles of the oral cavity. The conscientious dentist will examine the nasopharynx and the larynx and look for lesions on the face and extremities. Diagnostic capabilities are becoming more comprehensive than in the past.

Emphasis on symptomatic treatment is being modified as the dentist becomes cognizant of the chronicity of the dental diseases and becomes alert to sores, hoarseness, pain, and other possible indications of oral and perioral cancer. Using this approach, the modern dentist is concerned with the whole person. In the care of the aged and the very young, for example, there is a new emphasis on nutrition and its role in oral health.[11] There is also increased interaction with other members of the health professions, a notable example being the effort of dentists, pediatricians, and pharmacists to eliminate the use of tetracycline during the development of dentition because the drug causes unsightly staining of the teeth. Dental students and faculty at the University of Washington are developing an interdisciplinary course on "preventive practices in pediatric health." Participating students are from nursing, home economics (dietetics), and dentistry.

There is a concern today for protecting the dental patient from secondary injury and the untoward medical sequelae of dental treatment. A significant number of injuries have resulted from dental therapy.[12] Followup treatment is a major concern, reflecting the growing recognition that medical problems, such as postoperative infection with hepatitis type B, are sometimes associated with dental treatment.[19] Unfortunately, epidemiological studies which might help us to understand some of these general medical problems have not been done.* There are, however, several constructive examples of how dentists in some communities have responded to the expanded role expectation in regards to general medical problems. Dentists in New Jersey[1] have organized projects to study their role in the early diagnosis of hypertension and have demonstrated that routinely taking a patient's blood pressure can help detect preclinical cases. Presently, some dental schools[21] are providing clinical instruction for dental students in indirect laryngoscopy, making dentists capable of early detection of malignant changes.

The boundaries of dental responsibility in the diagnosis and management of systemic disease are not clearly defined, although there has been a great deal of speculation about the future stomatologist. Routine technical treatments are being delegated to auxiliary personnel, and dental educators are being encouraged to broaden the dentist's education. The minimal expectation today is that the dentist be able to detect the oral signs of systemic disease, diabetes, hypertension, and leukemia and to refer the patient to a physician or to another discipline for special care services.[15] In content, dentistry appears to be slowly approaching the status of a medical specialty with a greater respect for comprehensive health services. A few universities have initiated experimental joint D.D.S.-M.D. degree programs for dentists interested in medicine or medical research. The University of Washington, for example, has such a program in oral and maxillofacial surgery. The incorporation of additional medical instruction into the dental curriculum, especially in the area of physical diagnosis, is inevitable. It is unlikely, however, that designation as a medical specialty will be accepted in the near future, even if organized medicine were to accept a more integrated role for the dentist. Traditional practices are still quite apparent.

In this period of change from the traditional to a broader role for the dentist, it is inevitable that certain specific adverse outcomes will appear. Table 1, taken from our ongoing analysis of the end results of dental care, gives examples of how general medical problems can occur in dental treatment. Failure to take a medical history could result in a postoperative subacute bacterial endocarditis or greatly increase the likelihood that a diabetic patient may develop an infection. Postoperative infections, which can occur with errors in diagnosis, treatment, or followup, can be avoided by premedication with antibiotics. A symptom of Addison's disease in the mouth is pigmented gingiva, and the careful dentist would note such an abnormality in his examination.

Dental radiographic examination should be done so that pre-existing osseous lesions caused by infection will be diagnosed. Lack of skill in oral surgery may result in poor management of a fracture with the consequence of an osteomyelitis. Unconventional treatments such as metal denture frameworks implanted in the jaw

---

*Since this communication was originally submitted, an outbreak of hepatitis transmitted by dental personnel to 13 patients has been reported.[24] One dentist returned to practice after eight months of convalescence, but while still HB Ag-positive. Patients developed the symptoms of the disease three months later.

TABLE 1. Errors in the medical component of dental care with a high degree of avoidability

Avoidable event: Postoperative infection

Process	Examples
Adverse outcomes from errors in diagnosis	Errors in taking patient history resulting in postoperative subacute bacterial endocarditis. Failure to diagnose a pre-existing osteomyelitis.
Adverse outcomes from errors in treatment	Lack of skill and poor management of a fracture resulting in osteomyelitis. Infection from unconventional treatment such as implanted denture frameworks. Antral infection from tooth root pushed into sinus.
Adverse general medical outcomes	Septicemia from unsterile needles. Superinfection from inadequate dose of antibiotic. Serum hepatitis from unsterile instruments. Dry socket (osteitis) from unsterile extraction instruments. Tetanus infection after replanatation of an avulsed tooth without active prophylaxis.
Adverse outcomes from errors in followup	Delay in prescribing antibiotics for postoperative septic cellulitis causing unnecessary surgery. Failure to follow up and treat with antibiotics fungal infection in patient.
Adverse outcomes from legally proscribed acts	Abandonment or failure to treat symptomatic patient postoperatively.

may provide pathways for microorganisms from the oral cavity into the mandible, causing severe infection. Other examples found in the malpractice literature are septicemia from the use of unsterilized needles and serum hepatitis resulting postoperatively from the use of unsterilized cutting instruments. Most of these adverse conditions could be avoided by the use of presterilized disposable materials. There are other examples in the literature of a failure or delay in prescribing antibiotics for a postoperative cellulitis which resulted in major injury and disfigurement.

The 1971 Survey of Dental Practice by the American Dental Association[2] asked dentists about their provision of lead protection aprons for patients during exposure to dental radiographs. Fifty-two per cent reported that they used leaded aprons in practice, yet only 26.7 per cent did so for all patients. Almost 60 per cent of younger dentists (under 40) used protective aprons; older dentists used the devices much less regularly. These practices represent at the very least an insensitivity to the possible medical complications from the increasing use of x-rays in this country.

The medical problems encountered by dentists are not surprising, and they clearly indicate that decisive action by educators, practitioners, and state regulatory officials is needed. Dental schools must begin to make serious provisions for re-educating both clinical faculties and community dentists since the vast majority of clinicians have not received advanced education in these areas. They need to be brought up-to-date in regard to their new role of providing broad medical services as part of general dentistry. Studies of the effectiveness of continuing education in dentistry[9] (and medicine as well[16]) have shown little relation between course work and subsequent improvement in practice standards. In general, continuing dental education is didactic rather than participatory and more oriented toward practice management than toward broad medical responsibility. A number of researchers[20] have studied efforts to induce dental practitioners to do better examinations for oral cancer and to increase their use of oral pathology laboratories for instructional and practice purposes. Each of these efforts has been unsuccessful, as evidenced by the high mortality rate for oral cancer.[21]

State boards of dental examiners must take a more effective role in protecting the public. In particular, boards of examiners should begin to identify adverse and avoidable outcomes of dental treatment, such as the postoperative infections described above, and should design reporting systems to monitor unfavorable consequences. Peer review committees must begin to sanction and mandate specific kinds of remedial training for dentists whose standards are obsolete. The alternative, it appears, will be a tendency by patients to sue the dentist.[8] During the next several years, dentists will have little involvement with Professional Standards Review Organizations (PSRO), since the major orientation of the PSRO initially will be toward more effective management of hospitalized patients and dental care is primarily ambulatory and furnished in private offices. Much profile data and a greatly improved record keeping method are needed before the quality of dental care can be efficiently monitored.

Thus a hidden but most important facet of dental service is its medical component. This chapter has identified some of the many factors involved in the evolution of rigorous standards for dentists in the incorporation of general medical services into their practice and has delineated areas in which these changes are occurring. Avoidable adverse outcomes in the dental office have been highlighted to stress the importance of establishing quality standards of dental care for the protection of the public during this transitional period as dentists adapt to new areas of responsibility and role changes.

REFERENCES

1.   Berman, Charles L.: Screening by dentists for hypertension. N. Engl. J. Med. 290:579, 1974.
2.   Bureau of Economic Research and Statistics: The 1971 Survey of Dental Practice. American Dental Association, Chicago, 1972, pp. 48-49.
3.   Cole, R. B., and Cohen, L. K.: Dental manpower: Estimating resources and requirements. Milbank Mem. Fund Q. XLIX (3), Part 2, pp. 29-62, July 1971.
4.   Current Estimates from the Health Interview Survey: Vital and Health Statistics. Series 10, number 79, DHEW(HSM) 73-1505, Table 19. (Number of percent distribution of persons by time interval since last dental visit according to sex and age. United States, 1971.)

5. Denenberg, H. S.: A Shopper's Guide to Dentistry. Pennsylvania Insurance Department, Harrisburg, 1973.

6. Friedman, Jay W.: Dentistry in the geriatric patient. Geriatrics 23:98, 1968.

7. Goulding, P. C.: What the public thinks of the dentist and dental health. J. Am. Dent. Assoc. 70:1211, 1965.

8. Himmelfarb, Robert: The professional liability committee—first line of defense in malpractice claims. J. Am. Dent. Assoc. 88:341, 1974.

9. Hozid, J. L.: Role of continuing education in dental obsolescence. J. Am. Dent. Assoc. 79:1299, 1969.

10. Ingle, J.: American dental care—1972: A plan designed to deliver preventive and therapeutic dental care to the children of America. Presented at the Conference of Dental Examiners and Dental Educators, Chicago, Illinois, Feb. 11-12, 1972.

11. Katz, Simon, McDonald, James L., Jr., and Stookey, George K.: Preventive Dentistry in Action. D.C.P. Publishing, Indiana University Foundation, Upper Montclair, N.J., 1972, pp. 205-240.

12. Louisell, D.W., and Williams, H.: Medical Malpractice. M. Bender, New York, 1972, Vol. II; and 1973 Supplement to Appendix A.

13. Medical Care Costs and Prices. Background Book, DHEW(SSA) 72-11908. Office of Research and Statistics, Jan. 1972, p. 52.

14. Milgrom, Peter: Continuing education and prospective for national standard of dental care. J. Dent. Educ. 38:482, 1974.

15. Milgrom, Peter, Nash, Jon, and Rovin, Sheldon: Identifying leadership careers in the dental profession. J. Dent. Educ. 38:106, 1974.

16. Miller, G. E.: Continuing education for what? J. Med. Educ. 42:320, 1967.

17. Millis, John S.: The future of health care. The role of the consumer. J. Am. Soc. Prevent. Dent. 2:11, 1972.

18. Moen, B. D.: Deficiencies in knowledge attitudes and behavior which make public dental education necessary. American Dental Association, Bureau of Economic Research and Statistics, Chicago, 1960, mimeographed.

19. Personal Communication: Letter from Valerie Hurst, Ph.D., to Peter M. Milgrom, D.D.S., May 2, 1974, including Resolution 9-74-H of the House of Delegates of the American Association of Dental Schools concerning sterilization of dental instruments.

20. Ryan, R. M.: Continuing education research, in Richards, N.D., and Cohen, L. K. (Eds.): Social Sciences and Dentistry; A Critical Bibliography. A. Sijthoff, The Hague, 1971.

21. Sabes, William R., and Eversole, L. R.: The dentist's role in the detection of laryngeal and nasopharyngeal lesions: Prevention of morbidity. J. Am. Soc. Prevent. Dent. 4:36, 1974.

22. Sarner, Harvey: Dental Jurisprudence. W. B. Saunders Co., Philadelphia, 1963, pp. 32-45.

23. Strickland, Stephen P.: U.S. Health Care: What's Wrong and What's Right. Universe Books, New York, 1972, pp. 100-102.

24. Levin, Michael L.: Hepatitis B transmission by dentists. J.A.M.A. 228:1139, 1974.

Private Nursing Practice:
Some Facilitators and Barriers
in Health Care

NANCY S. KELLER, R.N., Ph.D.

One of the major assumptions that supports the emergence of the private practice of nursing and the evolution of the "extended-expanded" role concept involves considerations of efficiency and economy. Presumably nurses in private practice can deliver certain kinds of health care services more directly, with less cost to clients, and with coincident higher levels of consumer satisfaction than does our present health care delivery system. But even though I had been active in nursing for almost 15 years before entering private practice, it was difficult to predict the lessons to be learned about the interrelationships among care, cost, and consumer satisfaction from the private practice perspective and mode of providing nursing service.

It was clear, however, from my previous nursing experience that underlying the primary problems in nursing were issues of visibility and manpower.[4] Professional nurses who work in complex organizations usually form relationships with patients who have one or more primary ties to physicians or to the institution—be it hospital, clinic, or home health agency. For these nurses, interactions with patients are somewhat dependent on physicians, and nurses do not (nor do the traditional role relationships readily permit them much latitude to) present themselves as independent contractors for providing distinctly separate and visible nursing services. Within programs of education, continued emphasis on preparing nurses for middle-management positions will further diminish the visibility of nurses' work for direct evaluation by patients.

The second issue, manpower, has become more evident as government and insurance carriers attempt to equalize accessibility to the present health care delivery system and assure high quality services at reasonable cost. Nurse practitioners (in contrast to physician's assistants) are employed as primary personnel to increase the number of persons who enter the health care delivery system, hopefully at a more

37

appropriate time and place for entry. Nurses are expected to identify needs, and through nurses' efforts in this new role, more and more patient and system needs have been identified. The impact is that the system must adapt to delivering a greater amount of units of service to meet the increased demand. Unfortunately, emphasis has remained on the delivery of services at the expense of consumer education in utilization of these services. Nurses who contend that one of the major deficiencies of the present health care system is the number of people who do not have easy access to it are automatically ascribing to a basic quantitative premise, i.e., the number of people left out of the system need attention and service. However, one questions the quality of care in a system that, for example, identifies a client's need for assistance in walking, delivers a walker to the client's home, but does not instruct the client as to the use of the walker. Why should we register surprise when we hear that the person still falls when trying to get around her home?

These two issues provided the cornerstone of thought for me concerning the quality of services presently being delivered *and* nursing's responsibility to do something about it. The profession of nursing is alive with alternative philosophical approaches to the issues. The continuing controversy offers rallying points for professional organization and unification of references for curricula and acts as a springboard from which new models of nursing practice are launched, but the underlying issues still need further explication and study.

When nurses assume new roles and tasks in the attempt to deliver more services to more people, they are viewed too frequently as "filling the gap," as "the physician's handmaidens," and are also accused of delivering "second-class medical care."[5] These implicit or explicit accusations are attitudinal barriers to practice. The truth is that there are many well-prepared nurses providing high quality nursing services that are not yet publically recognized.

The problems for nurse practitioners (especially those who hang out their own shingles) arise from duplication of health care services and from some of the legal and ethical ties to the professional practice of medicine. Any nurse in private practice quickly learns the impact of certain barriers to her (his) capabilities in providing diagnostic and prescriptive services. The lack of physician referrals and lack of third party payments to nurses[1] are two definite barriers to private nursing practice and complicate the means by which clients can enter and leave most health care systems.

From the outset, I have been less concerned with the provision of more medical care services to the public than with the public's need for a kind of care that provides more and different kinds of information and emphasizes learning how to make use of the prescribed treatment modalities. It seems to me that consumers often received little or no information that helps them feel in command of themselves and certain situations. All too frequently, explanations given to clients are technical and procedural rather than descriptive of what the patient might experience. That is, instead of telling the patient what is going to happen to him, he is told what others are going to do to him. By describing the event in terms of the provider, we leave the patient with any number of unanswered questions.

Essentially, I have been less interested in becoming a "physician-extender" and more interested in becoming a "client-extender." Just as a professional or paraprofessional enlarges the influence of a physician when she or he assumes a physician-extender role, so does a client-extender enlarge the influence of the client. Just as physicians have some tasks that can be delegated to trained persons, clients have some tasks that can be done as well or better by others, e.g., obtaining accurate information, ascertaining options, and comparing differing advice. Being a client-extender means: (1) taking the client's position and perceptions as givens; (2) negotiating with the client concerning delegation of certain tasks that the nurse will do with and for him; and (3) helping the client use his own power to maintain control over certain aspects of the management of his health problem. The client-extender's primary relationship is with the client, just as the physician-extender's is with the physician.

A recent description of clients' informational needs suggests the concept of an "information broker."[2] This concept encompasses many of the activities that form the content of the client-extender role for nurses; in short, to work consistently at providing options and accurate information and at verifying or correcting the client's impressions. Either term (client-extender or information broker) certainly is a more accurate label than "patient advocate" if one believes that clients who have the necessary information and capabilities can state their own case and plead their own cause. Only when that capability is lacking does a client-extender take over the delegated task.

With the client-extender concept in mind, another nurse and I began private practice. We used Henderson's philosophy of nursing since we wanted to offer clients the knowledge and skills of nursing that would help extend the client's own knowledge, strength, and influence while ill or while trying to maintain or improve his health status.[3] This philosophy has helped us learn a great deal about the capabilities of clients and about ways to facilitate their care amid the many barriers in our present health care delivery system.

Clients who came to us during the past year were primarily concerned about a void they had perceived in the medical care system, specifically the unwillingness of physicians to answer their questions about treatment modalities and about choosing one treatment in favor of another. Most clients were not too critical of the quality of medical care, but many did not understand the rationale for medical decisions and prescriptions. They seemed to trust the efficacy of the treatment physicians prescribed, but they were critical of the physician's manner and attitudes toward them. Most importantly, the clients were concerned about not being allowed to participate in decisions about their own care. These barriers to care have been eliminated in our private nursing practices.

Since most of our clients were over 65 and hypertensive, they had problems of chronic disability and fixed income. Our clients expressed dissatisfaction with (1) the long waiting periods before the nurse took their blood pressure, (2) the physician saying so little (even if he also took the client's blood pressure), other than comments such as, "Keep taking your pills and I'll see you again in three months," and (3) paying as much as $8.00 to $15.00 for an office visit to the physician. These clients realized the potential hazards of uncontrolled elevated blood pressures, and they knew that the physician's prescribed medications would decrease their blood pressures—even though they did not like the side effects of the medications.

It became evident that nurses in private practice could remedy these three dominant client dissatisfactions. To begin with, we were able to take the client's blood pressure soon after arrival at our office. We encouraged clients to tell us about themselves and what they knew about their patterns of elevated blood pressure. And finally, we set a reasonable fee for taking blood pressures, which was from $2.00 to $5.00, depending upon the client's age and ability to pay.

Much to our relief, the clients were the first to recognize that visits to a nurse were *not* substitutes for visits to a physician. Clients repeated their realistic appreciation of their medical care, but also said that they no longer expected the kind of care they had previously desired from physicians since they now had it from professional nurses. It is interesting to note that they might have continued to seek this supportive-informative care from physicians had their real need for this kind of health service not been provided for by nurses or others.

In general, we found that clients wanted their blood pressure checked and wanted some information, verification, and corrective feedback from a health professional when they thought their health status was in potential danger. While we might have spent time teaching them about what blood pressure is, what the measurements mean, and how the levels are evaluated by the American Heart Association, our clients preferred a very simple kind of feedback on whether or not their blood pressure had changed. Clients tried to correlate their blood pressure readings with daily activities and events. The service these hypertensive patients wanted and which we believe has improved the quality of their care had to do with matching life situations with bodily sensations related to changes in blood pressure. More specifically, the client wanted some reliable indication about whether his blood pressure was high enough to merit concern and a trip to the physician.

Obviously, the client can afford several blood pressure checks between visits to his physician. He can check his hypotheses about what makes his blood pressure rise or fall, and he can verify or correct his knowledge about his body and his reactions to stress. The client visited us whenever he thought that his blood pressure was changing. One might think that these clients worried unduly about every fluctuation in their blood pressure, but this was not the case. Some clients told us that their physicians made them feel "neurotic" about their concern with the level of their blood pressure between visits to the doctor. Most clients averaged one or two visits to us each month, and we found that their concerns were legitimate, rational, and clearly relevant.

One thing that became evident as we interacted with clients was our own discomfort with redirecting client behavior beyond the medical model expectations. We found it was easy and a natural response to tell clients, "You ought to take the pills your doctor ordered," or "You need to see your physician about the elevation in your blood pressure." But these statements (appropriate as they might be in some instances) did not support or reinforce the reasons clients were choosing to come to nurses rather than to physicians. Instead, we learned to respond to the clients' concerns and needs with the supportive care that nurses can provide.

When we directed clients to seek medical advice when their blood pressure warranted it, we also provided the physician with a profile of changes in blood pressure readings taken between the physician visits. At each visit, the client's blood pressure was taken and compared with previous readings, past experiences, and his bodily sensations, thereby obtaining a fairly complete profile for each client. When events or concerns known to precipitate a rise or fall in blood pressure occurred, anticipated or not, the client was directed to return for blood pressure checks as soon as the impact of the event was realized. The client was also encouraged to determine what events had an impact on his blood pressure.

As nurses, we also focused upon the client's rationale for taking or *not* taking prescribed anti-hypertension medication. The clients have freely admitted abuses of medication. They believe that if one pill is good, then two or three will be better. They also believed that as soon as the blood pressure went down they were better and would conclude, "I don't need to take any more pills unless the pressure goes up again." Many believed that once the medication reduces the blood pressure it will not rise again soon, if at all. This accounts for their use of the word "unless" instead of "until" the pressure goes up again. Clients put a high value upon controlling their blood pressures by changing something about themselves or their life styles rather than by taking medication. Many of our clients did not want to take any medication, including aspirin. There were those who did not experience the cardinal symptoms of elevated blood pressure, and they found the side effects of prescribed medications objectionable. The paradox was that the disorder caused no specific discomfort, but the treatment did. It is no wonder that these clients tend to "cheat" on the medical regime.

A service appropriate to confronting this deficiency in medical management employed the knowledge and skills of clinical pharmacists. One effective directive statement by the nurse has been: "When you come in next time, we will talk with our clinical pharmacist about your specific medications." The nurse and clinical pharmacist as co-leaders of the next interview session give the client a "drug profile," that is, a description of the side effects of all the medications he takes (both prescribed and patent). The client receives a copy of this drug profile, directions for eliminating certain foods or beverages from his diet, and any other suggestions for diminishing side effects. Once the client is informed about the potential and real effects of the medications he is taking, we discuss the chronicity of hypertension with the client. We want clients to be free of excessive worry if and when the prescribed medication is inadequate in controlling their blood pressure with minimal side effects. We then discuss options for behavior modification that are feasible in terms of the data we have on causes of change in the client's blood pressure.

These kinds of repeated nurse-client interactions with hypertensive clients have led to the initiation of a health education program for persons who have, or fear they will have, high blood pressure. Small group sessions with nurses and clinical pharmacists as co-leaders give clients a structured opportunity to share common problems and respond to corrective feedback about decisions they must make in daily living.

The kinds of services that have emerged as a consequence of an open and sensitive client-centered approach have had several distinct values in facilitating the care of clients with hypertention. These nursing care modalities are different from those provided by physician-extender or physician practice. Nurse practitioners are being prepared to assess the efficacy of medications and to adjust dosages according to blood pressure readings. Our practice, however, is congruent with the client-extender position, in that we are providing the client with specific information and helping him with the task of processing that information into *options* that are acceptable within his life style and are anticipitory of daily life events.

To date, we have worked with 60 clients and find that very few have need of an advocate to request services for them within the second health care delivery system. Our clients do relate frustrations when they perceive a lack of response to their requests. Thus, in our private practice we have worked to strengthen the clients' capabilities to act as their own advocates through a kind of training in assertiveness. The clients had previously felt that their physicians *did not listen* to their accounts of what they thought was the problem and what they thought would or would not help them. Nurses, however, were valued for their capacity to listen, empathize, and care about the person in need. Once the nurse makes it her business to listen, to sift and sort out the data for meanings with the full participation of the client, and to verify the legitimate requests of other health workers, then the client is ready to assume more control over obtaining services for his needs. Using role rehearsals, the client was encouraged to rehearse his position confidently and to be able to sustain his position in the face of counter-positions when he knows his position is best for his own health and daily needs. In general, we found that once the client was given *and* helped to utilize information within his structure of meaning, he was ready to act as his own advocate for obtaining what help he needed.

An important change is being made when nurses say, "Tell your doctor," rather than only, "Listen to the doctor." The emphasis reinforces the client's role in giving information rather than only receiving it from the physician. Clients value the delineation of priorities in what to tell the physician and of options that are negotiable as a breakthrough in consumer power. Clients register surprise and satisfaction with the expectation that they can participate in (1) the request for information from physicians and other health workers via an authorization for release of information; (2) the formulation of summaries of information received from physicians; and (3) an open discussion and critique of information received from physicians. Client response has shown us that persons in need want to be treated as though the ultimate responsibility for their problems is their own. They simply want help to help themselves by some reminder that they do know how or can learn how to control some of the necessary aspects of the problem. This is a tremendously important *facilitation* process in supporting clients' rights and meeting their health needs.

Nurses in private practice must contend with traditional nurse-doctor relationships that loom as *barriers* to building a successful autonomous practice. At the time our office opened, we talked one-to-one with 15 separate physicians. Each physician was pleasant and interested in a description of our services. They wanted to know what *we nurses* could do that others in the community would or could not do. As we explained our services, the physicians would nod in assent and validate their understanding by giving us a case description to see if and how we would be able to *assist* the patient and the physician. At the close of these meetings, the physician would thank us for the information and say: "I think I can use you; I'll refer some of my patients to you." To date, we have not had a single physician referral. This fact is indicative of some of the interprofessional attitudinal barriers that limit health care services to people.

Some associates speculate that physicians do not give referrals because losing a single patient's call will reduce his income. This might well be true *if* other health workers are duplicating physician services and thereby competing for the same clients. This, however, does not appear to be the case, since clients are seeing their physicians regularly even when consulting other health professionals. But the encouraging fact that the client is learning how to evaluate health care services for himself could translate into an economic factor as the client decides, "No, I don't want that test done yet," or "No, I don't want to have surgery."

It is also probable that local physicians are not referring patients to us because they think we are practicing in the extended role even though we are not and have told them we are not. Duplication of diagnostic services external to the regulation of medicine is suspect and threatening. Local physicians did request that the State Board of Medical Examiners investigate our practice to ascertain if we were practicing medicine. Concurrently, an officer of the local medical society wrote to the State Board of Nurse Examiners registering the concern that we might not be practicing nursing according to the law. The Medical Board's investigator, after seeing the complete absence of examining tables or other medical equipment in our office, admitted he did not know what questions to ask. He tape-recorded our comments about the services being provided and left with the remark that if we were found to be doing something wrong, we would receive a letter from the Board telling us to cease and desist the specified activities. If there was nothing wrong, however, we would hear nothing—and would not even receive a notice that the Board had reviewed the information and found us without flaw. To date, almost eight months after the investigation, we have heard nothing. The inquiry to the State Board of Nurse Examiners about our violation of the nurse practice act did not go unanswered; an official letter from the Nurse Board fully explicated the differences in practicing nursing *in* and *out* of the extended role.

Investigatory power and withholding of referral when nurse-provided services could much improve quality of care are activities in the politics of intimidation and are barriers to the full utilization of nursing skills. Passive-agressive responses to the private practice of nursing are just as frustrating. Our requests to speak to the medical society or its officers and to officially inform the local medical community of our services have been consistently ignored and unacknowledged.

Such experiences as the above remind nurses that the more viable and facilitating forms of private practice are likely to be those linked directly to client needs and only indirectly to medical practitioners. Moreover, we have found that by utilizing the client's own physician(s) and making appropriate requests for information and direction for our activities, we are beginning to "co-opt" a few physicians who believe that nursing services delivered from our model of private practice are complemental to theirs and generally supportive to the efforts of all persons involved. These same physicians are more apt to refer other patients to us. In the meantime, the lack of immediately available physician support is a factor that impedes the development of nursing's private practice. One can readily appreciate the fact that it takes a large volume of cases at $2.00 to $5.00 or even $15.00 to $30.00 per visit to financially support nurses in solo, let alone in group practice. The greater proportion of the income necessary to support my partner and I comes from working as what we call "nurse-extenders." As we are employed by directors of nursing for consultation and staff development programs in local hospitals, nursing homes, and health department, we are extending the influence of a nursing perspective in these agencies. This perspective contrasts with those perspectives formerly dominant, when nursing directors had only medical, management, and systems analysis professionals as consultants, with relatively little access to nursing consultants.

Our preference has been to capitalize on the full array of our separate and collective talents, education, and experience in order to create markets for research and consultation, rather than to practice only part time, which is the apparent choice and advice of a number of nurses who have tried private practice.[1] Part-time effort with this new experiment in nursing is yet another factor that restricts the volume and diversity of practice and its economic benefits. It is true that we have developed some models of private practice that have demonstrated an improved quality of care with a reasonable cost, quicker accessibility, and noteworthy client satisfactions, but other modes and sources of health care are being devised by government, medicine, and business interests[4] that have the power to command more resources and public recognition than nursing can. Hopefully, more nursing practices will be based on enough diversity of services so as to financially and professionally support the private practice of nursing with its tremendous potential to meet client needs.

We have learned some important lessons about the complexity of health care delivery if we learn to place emphasis on: (1) describing attributes and characteristics of the system where consumers now find deficiencies; (2) ascertaining what services would provide or reinforce this qualitative aspect of the system; (3) deciding whether these services can be provided by nurses; and (4) sharing this information among members of the nursing profession.

This process is as simple as starting with the problems that clients bring to nurses and the things clients expect nurses to perform without direction from other health professionals. The real way to discover nursing's unique contributions to health care is *not* through constant debates and harangues among ourselves, but rather by grounding our contribution in a value or sets of values that are naturally reinforced when we care for clients, in our dependence upon clients to bring certain of their needs to us, and in their dependence on us to provide certain services.

We will discover nursing's unique contributions by increasing the visibility and accessibility of nurses (independent of former associations with hospitals, clinics, physicians' offices, etc.), so that the public learns to identify nursing skills among the myriad tasks and skills found in hospitals, clinics, and so on. The paradox that will be discovered by nurses who try private practice is that by being separate and distinct in terms of accessibility, there is a greater sense of interdependence among nurses, clients, and other health professionals. Interdependence is the key concept, reducing the focus on nurses attainment of independence.

While private practice has helped us to see more clearly many barriers and facilitators to health care delivery, it has also had some disappointments. However, its promise and potential for contributing to health care are strong incentives to continue to explore the relationships among the quality and cost of care, client satisfaction, and the significant role of the nurse in health care delivery services. In our assessment, the potentials far outweigh the obstacles in providing quality *nursing* care through the methods and modes of private nursing practice.

REFERENCES

1. Agree, B. C.: Beginning an independent nursing practice. American Journal of Nursing 74:636, April 1974.
2. Annas, G. J., and Healy, J.: The Patient Rights Advocate. Paper presented at Symposium (The Rights of Patients and Their Providers) sponsored by Boston College Law School-Tufts Medical School Joint Center for the Study of Law, Medicine, and the Life Sciences, April 19, 1973. (To be published in the Journal of Nursing Administration.)
3. Harmer, B., and Henderson, V.: Textbook of the Principles and Practice of Nursing, ed. 5. The Macmillan Company, New York, 1955.
4. Keller, N. S.: The Nurses' role: Is it expanding or shrinking? Nursing Outlook. 21:236, April 1973.
5. Lublin, J. S.: Supernurses Provide Care for Thousands, Helping Doctors Cope. The Wall Street Journal XCI, July 3, 1974.

Current Public Policy and Medical Care Evaluation

JAMES J. McCORMACK, Ph.D.

INTRODUCTION

The development of public health policy has been traditionally characterized by concern for specific population groups, such as disabled persons, infants and children, and low-income women of child-bearing age. Emphasis has been placed upon the design of special programs to assure the accessibility and availability of health care services to these groups. There has been, however, a dramatic change in the nature of public debate regarding health care policy in the last few years. This change completes a full circle in the debate that began with reports in the early 1930s advocating large-scale restructuring of the health delivery system, then the call for enactment of incremental provisions to improve health care for disadvantaged populations, and now again calls are heard for wholesale restructuring of the relationships among the various components of the health care system: consumers, providers, payers, and regulators.

Contemporary health policy analyses invariably take note of two major issues: (1) the significance of rising medical care costs and the percentage of the gross national product relegated to health and (2) the increasing proportion of health expenditures financed through the public sector. These basic socio-economic and political facts form a familiar platform for those who argue for greater consolidation and reorganization of the components of the health care industry to permit the application of modern-day planning and management techniques of control and forecasting. In these proposals, a significant shift in the balance of power from practitioners and providers to those who finance and regulate health care services can be identified.[1]

The American public has been subjected to a barrage of information from elected officials, economists, and other opinion leaders that indicates a contemporary health care "crisis" demanding the highest possible national priority. Legislation has been prepared to establish federal grant programs to foster various types of prepaid group practice corporations. National health insurance proposals have been written and rewritten setting forth a series of different tactics and provisions designed to remedy all manners of deficiencies attributed to present arrangements. Approximately a dozen national health insurance bills will be introduced in the Congress this year. Eilers and Moyerman[2] give an in-depth presentation of the issues and problems related to national health insurance public policy.

Experience with the Medicare and Medicaid programs has had a great influence on the formation of the present agenda for public discussion about health care policies for the United States. Problems of planning, administration, and control have contributed to the high costs of both programs. The Medicare and Medicaid programs were instituted in a market environment in which there were insufficient organizational links between the various components of the health care industry and where the probable effect of this large infusion of dollars into the industry was not clearly understood. In addition, utilization review functions have not been carried out as intended by the provisions of the authorizing legislation.[3]

Quality control of health care has emerged as an important issue in discussions regarding reorganization and restructuring the health care system. As Kissick and Martin have noted,[1] with the rapid growth of the health industry, its subsequent institutionalization, and increased public payments, the subjective assessments made by individual practitioners no longer constitute a viable response to quality control requirements. Persons are now cared for by multiple types of health care practitioners, each of whom must have some role in quality and cost of control.

A growing number of observers, who discuss the assessment of quality in health care services in terms of the familiar Donabedian triad of structure, process, and outcome,[4-6] point out that increased public funding of health services will require a more visible and organized system of quality control to meet increased expectations of public accountability.

Regulation of the quality of health care has been addressed in two recent major legislative efforts with the purpose of defining and creating systematic national programs for quality and cost controls. The 1972 Amendments to the Social Security Act (PL 92-603, Section 249F) require establishment of Professional Standards Review Organizations (PSRO) to monitor health care services financed by three public programs: Medicare, Medicaid, and Maternal and Child Health Services. The Health Maintenance Organization Act of 1973 (H.R. 93-222) supports the development of prepaid group practice organizations. The promotion of the health maintenance organization (HMO) concept has greatly depended upon the claim of a higher quality of health care at lower costs in comparison with the traditional fee-for-service arrangements.[7] The HMO legislation contains major provisions that bear upon the regulation of health care quality.

Selected aspects of these two bills are reviewed in the following two sections. Their probable contributions to public regulation of health care quality are examined in the concluding summary.

HEALTH MAINTENANCE ORGANIZATION ACT OF 1973

Public documents dealing with national health policy have increasingly made reference to the desirability of constructing a more efficient and effective health service delivery system. Presidential commissions and experts within and outside of the government have noted that continued reliance upon the present complex array of medical services is a questionable policy if the country is to pursue the goal of making high quality health care available to all.[8,9]

A different arrangement of relationships between medical care providers, financers, and consumers is considered necessary by many health policy analysts. Since 1970, the phrase "health maintenance organization" has come to symbolize this search for a new system of health services delivery. The phrase is operationally defined to mean a network of services under a central direction that is available to a defined population and financed with prepaid per capita payments. Referring to various studies, many analysts have sought to construct a case for the reorganization of the present arrangements through which medical care services are made available.[10-12] The federal government's influence on the structure and organization of the health industry increased with the enactment of the recent HMO legislation.[13]

Analysts concerned with the interaction between the medical care provider complex and the consumer public have noted that a medical care system must be developed in which services are made more accessible, continuous, and responsive to consumer needs. Roemer[14] has noted that the goal of universally available quality health care at acceptable costs involves three subgoals or objectives: promotion of quality care, achievement of accessibility to care for all, and establishment of control over costs. This view seems widely shared.[15,16]

Federal subsidy for the development and initial operation of health maintenance organizations is a tactic designed for further progress toward the three objectives noted by Roemer. Much of the argument for enacting this legislation that provides incentives for the reorganization of health services delivery has centered around presumed economic efficiency and methods for controlling the costs of delivering care.[17]

Accessibility to care for all has two major aspects: financial accessibility and resource distribution. Financial barriers to care must await the development of a national health insurance for a reduction to their absolute minimum. The new HMO legislation addresses the distribution of resources and requires that any application for planning, developmental, or operational support must include medically underserved urban or rural groups within its enrollment area. The legislation also specifies that not less than 20 per cent of the sums appropriated in any fiscal year be allocated for projects that may reasonably be expected to have two-thirds of their membership drawn from residents of nonmetropolitan areas.

While this legislation includes sections related to achieving accessibility and establishing cost control, attention is focused upon the promotion of quality health care and must be recognized as a major federal initiative on this issue. The bill authorizes a $10 million appropriation for an extensive study, the Health Care

Quality Assurance Programs Study, that would form the basis for establishing specifications "for an effective quality assurance system."[18] The bill requires the Secretary of Health, Education, and Welfare (HEW) to enter into a contract for this study within 90 days of enactment and delegates responsibility for a tight reign on the design and conduct of the study to the Congress. It provides that the study be conducted by a nonprofit private organization and that the plan for the study be submitted by the contractor to the Committee on Interstate and Foreign Commerce of the House of Representatives and to the Committee on Labor and Public Welfare of the Senate by June 30, 1974; a final report is to be submitted to Congress by January 31, 1976. The proposed study has a very broad sweep and is clearly viewed as a major means for establishing a definitive quality assurance system.

The following excerpt from the legislation defines elements of the Health Care Quality Assurance Programs Study:

Sec. 4. (a) The Secretary of Health, Education, and Welfare shall contract, in accordance with sub-section (b), for the conduct of a study to:

(1) analyze past and present mechanisms (both required by law and voluntary) to assure the quality of health care, identify the strengths and weaknesses of current major prototypes of health care quality assurance systems, and identify on a comparable basis the costs of such prototypes;

(2) provide a set of basic principles to be followed by any effective health care quality assurance system, including principles affecting the scope of the system, methods for assessing care, data requirements, specifications for the development of criteria and standards which relate to desired outcomes of care, and means for assessing the responsiveness of such care to the needs and perceptions of the consumers of such care;

(3) provide an assessment of programs for improving the performance of health practitioners and institutions in providing high quality health care, including a study of the effectiveness of sanctions and educational programs;

(4) define the specific needs for a program of research and evaluation in health care quality assurance methods, including the design of prospective evaluation protocols for health care quality assurance systems; and

(5) provide methods for assessing the quality of health care from the point of view of consumers of such care.[18]

This funded contract and the requirements for reporting to the health-related House and Senate committees represent the most intense involvement of elected public officials in quality control of health care to be found in any legislation in the United States. The dates set for completion of the study and submission of a report to the Congress indicate that the legislators desire a rapid analysis of present quality review arrangements and development of guidelines for a preferred system for a national program.

Other provisions of the HMO Act also underline the important concern for quality in the development of the HMO program. The manner of operation of a health maintenance organization is described under Section 1301, Subsection C[19] and indicates that each health maintenance organization shall institute procedures such that they are able to report on: (1) the cost of its operations; (2) the patterns of utilization of its services; (3) the availability, accessibility, and acceptability of its services; and (4) the developments in the health status of its clients. These requirements are consistent with the quality of care approach described in the discussion of Professional Standards Review Organizations below.

The consistantly high priority of quality assurance in HMO programs is also apparent in the requirements for applications for grants and contracts. The Secretary of HEW may not approve an application unless the applicant specifies an existing or anticipated arrangement for an ongoing quality assurance program. The Comptroller General is required to evaluate the operations of at least 50 of the HMOs for which assistance is provided after completion of 36 months of operation. The items to be addressed in the evaluation are specified in the legislation. It is further required that the Comptroller General and the Secretary of HEW both evaluate "the impact that health maintenance organizations, individually, by category, and as a group, have on the health of the public" for inclusion in their reports to Congress.[19]

In addition to the independent quality assurance programs study, the legislation provides funds to the Assistant Secretary for Health to conduct research and evaluation programs on quality assurance programs. The appropriations are for $4 million for fiscal year 1974, $8 million for 1975, $9 million for both 1976 and 1977, and $10 million for 1978. The Assistant Secretary must submit an annual report on these research and evaluation programs to both the President and the Congress concerning the quality of health care in the United States, the operation of quality assurance programs, and the advancements made in research and evaluation of the effectiveness, administration, and enforcement of quality assurance programs.

The required independent study may be viewed as a program of directed research since the elements of the study are specified in the legislation. The research and evaluation programs to be conducted by the Assistant Secretary for Health provide substantial sums for open-ended research and evaluation efforts. The HMO Act of 1973 proposes a total expenditure of $50 million for quality assurance studies through June 30, 1978.

PROFESSIONAL STANDARDS REVIEW ORGANIZATIONS

The evaluation of the quality and efficiency of services performed by physicians has traditionally been carried out by their peers and colleagues. The AMA explains peer review as an all-inclusive term for medical review efforts that include specific activities for institutional and ambulatory care evaluation. The scope of peer review in the lexicon of the medical profession incorporates inpatient hospital and extended care facility utilization review, medical audit, ambulatory care review, and claims review.[20] We will briefly review the position of organized medicine with regard to quality review before turning to the PSRO legislation.

Various local and state medical societies have fostered peer review efforts within institutions and at the community level under their aegis. These reviews are based upon consensually acceptable treatment modalities taken from available profiles of medical practice. Criteria are developed in the local community, used to identify deviancies, and reviewed by physicians within their own peer review program or as part of arrangements with some payer organization.[21]

Two main efforts fulfill medical society peer review responsibilities: medical practice analysis and medical care evaluation. Medical practice analysis requires the development and application of criteria for optimum medical care and evaluates the individual and the collective quality, volume, and the cost of medical care wherever provided. Medical care evaluation seeks to assure the quality of health care in a hospital or other health care institution and is viewed as "the educational function of the medical staff." Medical care evaluation is concerned with two dimensions of quality: (1) utilization review, the examination of the efficiency of the use of the institution, i.e., appropriateness of admissions, services ordered, length of stay, and discharge, and (2) medical audit, involving retrospective examinations of patient management with the goal of advancing the level of medical care through an educational process.

Thus the AMA concept of peer review includes a comprehensive requirement for review of resource utilization, appropriateness of clinical management practices, and attention to costs. In their preferred approach, responsibility is given to medical staffs within hospitals, community medical societies, and state medical associations to aid and assist in the coordination and development of review programs. The peer review manual indicates a clear preference for state medical associations as the primary sources of organizational and professional influence on the development of guidelines for quality review. However, the profession has not been successful in fostering well organized programs in all states. Development of state medical society programs reflecting the most desirable characteristics is incomplete and spotty.

The terms "peer review," "quality care assurance," and "professional standards review" have recently come into popular usage within the health policy arena. The American Medical Association, through its Council on Medical Services and its Committee on Health Care Financing, has sponsored regional and national conferences and workshops on peer review. The American Hospital Association and the Joint Commission on Accreditation of Hospitals have undertaken intensive projects to encourage more structured utilization review and medical audit programs within institutions. All of these national groups have participated in discussions on the formulation and operation of review efforts under Medicare (Title 18) and Medicaid (Title 19). As noted earlier, these review efforts have been ineffective and unsatisfactory. The reviews have focused on the use of institutional resources with respect to length of stay, and not upon medical audit issues of criteria for admission and standards of treatment, i.e., not on peer review or quality of care matters. The Social Security Amendments of 1972 (PL 92-603) contain provisions that permit the Secretary of HEW to require more effective utilization review procedures under Medicare and Medicaid. These procedures include precertification of all nonemergency admissions and specification of average permissible lengths of stay according to admitting diagnosis. Since two separate attempts to implement this pre-admission certification provision led to great uproars from medical and hospital interests, the provision was finally shelved by the Social Security Administration. Those who opposed the amendment held that it greatly prejudiced the development of the professional standards review organization concept. Since governmental strategy has generally stressed the responsibility of the medical profession for implementation of the PSRO legislation, the national program is considered a "last-ditch" effort to permit professionals to respond to the need for effective review through their own initiative before the demands of public accountability lead to an extensive government bureaucracy for quality review.

The public climate of concern about the "health care crisis" fostered legislative activity directed toward change in the structure and financing of health services. This building pressure led the American Medical Association to prepare a proposal for developing a national quality control program for public medical assistance programs. The AMA proposed that a Peer Review Organization (PRO) would establish a program whereby HEW would contract with state medical societies for the review of publicly supported health care. The state PRO would appoint local review panels which, in turn, could delegate their duties to existing review bodies.

While the AMA prefers PRO, it has accepted the PSRO as a law of the land. However, the AMA seeks to have the PSRO legislation amended to reflect some of its own concerns and preferences, particularly the establishment of authority at the state rather than local level.[23]

The Social Security Amendments of 1972 (Sec. 249F) provided for the establishment of Professional Standards Review Organizations consisting of 300 or more physicians in local areas. These locally-based PSROs are to assume the responsibility for comprehensive and ongoing review of services covered under the Medicare, Medicaid, and Maternal and Child Health (Title 5) programs. Local medical societies are given until January 1, 1976, to present physician-sponsored organizations for PSRO designation by the Secretary of HEW. The PSRO assumes the responsibility (with regard to the three federal programs mentioned) for assuring that institutional services are (1) medically necessary, (2) provided in accordance with professional standards, and (3) provided on an inpatient basis only when the appropriate services cannot effectively be provided on an outpatient basis or less expensively in an inpatient facility of a different type.[24] The law also provides that a PSRO, with the approval of the Secretary, may elect to assume responsibility for the review of noninstitutional care and other services provided under the three programs. The legislation makes it clear that the PSROs will not be involved with determinations of charges.

With the passage of the PSRO legislation, the Department of HEW established preliminary designations of 182 areas in which PSROs may be formed and provided a review period of approximately 90 days before publishing final area designations.[25] Following the final designation, the Secretary of HEW will make conditional designations of a PSRO for each area and may provide grants for assistance in the organization of these groups. The Act further provides that a PSRO will be identified for all areas by January 1, 1976. The legislation clearly indicates that the government desires the full cooperation of organized medicine at national, state, and local levels in the implementation of this program.[26] Federal officials seem to highly favor strengthening the traditional hospital-based medical audit and the development of PSRO approaches that are most acceptable to practicing physicians and osteopaths.

The organizational structure for implementation of the PSRO legislation includes establishment of an 11-member national Professional Standards Review Council, to which one osteopathic and ten medical doctors have been appointed. Members representing the American Medical Association, the American Hospital Association, the American Public Health Association, the National Medical Association, and the American Association of Foundation Medical Care Plans can be identified in addition to an advocate of prepaid closed panel group practice. A statewide Professional Standards Review Council is required in any state having three or more PSROs in operation. The actual review organizations, comprising approximately 180 areawide Professional Standards Review Organizations, will be incorporated nonprofit organizations independent of professional medical or osteopathic associations.

The responsibilities and functions of the PSROs are made explicit in Section 1155 of the legislation,[27] which specifically requires PSROs to take responsibility for precertification. They are provided the authority to determine, in advance, the medical necessity of elective hospital admissions, to determine whether Medicare or Medicaid shall pay for the care, and to make similar determinations with regard to any health care service which will consist of extended or costly treatment. It is required that profiles of care and services, both received and provided, be maintained and regularly reviewed. Physicians are excluded from review of hospitals in which they have active staff privileges. PSROs are permitted to utilize and accept the findings of existent review committees in the hospitals, providing that such review committees meet the standards of the local PSRO.

It is of interest that the tasks of establishing norms of care, diagnosis, and treatment are a responsibility of the local PSRO, though they must have final approval from the National Professional Standards Review Council. The National Council can thus be interpreted as the arbitrator of differences between local treatment norms in existence and those established as desirable for that given area.

The Act requires PSRO review to justify payment for services provided under the federal health care programs. Providers or practitioners may be excluded from eligibility to provide services on a reimbursable basis under the federal programs if any PSRO so recommends to the Secretary of HEW. Beneficiaries, whether recipients or providers, who disagree with the decision of the PSRO may appeal to the statewide PSRO and, if still dissatisfied, to the Secretary of HEW.

The National Professional Standards Review Council is required to submit to the Secretary of HEW and the Congress an annual report which must include comparative data on the results of review activities in each of the various PSRO areas.

The PSRO legislation did not specify amounts of appropriations to implement the program, but authorized the Secretary of HEW to pay expenses incurred from the federal Hospital Insurance Trust Fund, the federal Supplementary Medical Insurance Trust Fund, and from funds appropriated to the several health care programs under professional standards review.

The PSRO legislation has generally been criticized on two counts: that in-hospital services are overstressed[28] and that the initiative for review efforts is essentially a concern for cost control. However, considering the predictable difficulties in the implementation of this program, it seems reasonable that the initial task be limited to in-hospital care. The cost control issue did lead to action. In its report on the Medicare and Medicaid programs, the Senate Committee on Finance[29] expressed concern about dramatic cost increases and the lack of effective utilization controls in the programs, emphasizing the need for local independent organizations to assume responsibility for review of the services provided. The legislative response, however, has features similar to the PRO program of the American Medical Association and intends that the reviews will very certainly be consequential for quality as well as cost control. Of related interest here is the likelihood that other health care services for which professional review will be instituted would most immediately include those health practices having most significance within hospitals, e.g., nursing and pharmacy.

The governmental strategy for implementation of the PSRO law is quite different from that of the HMO bill. The former advocates a "go-slow" approach with an all-out effort to draw organized practitioners and health care institutions into a collaborative partnership to establish a national review system. The PSRO program will spend two to two and one-half years developing regulations for its conduct and administration.[30] Physicians in local areas will have considerable time to adjust their customary practices and arrangements to the slowly developing regional norms, criteria, and standards.

Farrell[30] provides the following definitions developed by the PSRO program regarding norms:

> Medical care appraisal norms are averages or medians of observed performance that are stated in numerical or statistical terms. Medical care criteria are a predetermined, measureable element of health care that are requisite to the delivery of care of high quality; they are developed by professionals relying on professional judgment, consensus, and expertise and on the professional literature. Standards are professionally developed measures of the range of acceptable variation from the norm or from criteria.

SUMMARY AND COMMENTARY

Responsibility for assuring service quality through self-regulation has been a definitional characteristic of groups wishing designation as a profession. Professional associations create codes of ethics and standards for training to guarantee the technical competence of their members. Among health professionals, all manners of societies attest to a certain practitioner's achievement of a superior skill in a specialized area. These certifications and recertifications are the most widespread response of various professions to the need for some type of minimal quality control and public accountability.

A growing number of health care workers carrying out activities in what might be considered the gray area between "occupation" and "profession" support the initiation of self-review and regulation. It would be interesting, though not appropriate in this review, to examine opposition to professional review among the more recently defined and less well established health care professions. I am not suggesting that the various health care professions are not interested in the quality of care rendered by their members but only pointing out that responses to public policy initiatives reflect organizational and identity needs often perceived to be quite different from those of the medical profession.

In recent years, organizations representing segments of the health care field have worked toward the design and dissemination of more objective experiential systems of public accountability in the area of peer review and quality assurance. Excellent examples of voluntarily initiated quality control programs are the American Medical Association's Peer Review system, the American Hospital Association's Quality Assurance Program, and the Trustee-Administrator-Physician Institutes on utilization review and medical audit of the Joint Commission on the Accreditation of Hospitals. Information systems to aid retrospective audits such as those of PAS-MAP and others also should be classed with these programs.

The time has come to acknowledge that these efforts have been either "too late" or "too little" to forestall public action. Sufficient success and visibility has not been demonstrated to forestall legislation regarding public regulation of health care quality, as evidenced by the PSRO amendment to the Social Security Act with its specific focus on review of quality of care. At this time, all indications point to the establishment of quality control through members of the profession whose activity is to be reviewed. Physicians and osteopaths are asked to band together to form local PSROs for peer review. Hospital utilization review committees are to be used wherever possible by the PSROs to avoid disruption of present arrangements and to build upon the work of the voluntary efforts previously mentioned. It seems likely that administrative guidelines will underscore this principle rather than construct alien new procedures to accomplish the aims of the legislation.

The decision to develop a review system as a collaborative venture of the government and the health care professions in what might be described as a quasi-voluntary organizational mode seems wise, but it would be foolhardy to maintain that if it does not work, the issue will be forgotten. It is more likely that a new organizational tactic less conciliatory toward organized professional groups would emerge.

The laissez faire strategy in developing the PSRO program contrasts sharply to the definitive requirements of the HMO legislation, which seeks to develop prescribed approaches to quality care measurement and assurance activities. It is logical to expect that the push provided in the HMO legislation and the eventual adoption of uniform review arrangements by HMOs will encourage PSROs to utilize products derived from HMO activities.

The $10 million Health Care Quality Assurance Programs Study of the HMO Act has the potential of becoming a bench mark study. The report very probably will initiate a major debate on the utility of various quality measurement programs affecting both publicly and privately supported payment arrangements. The final outcome may be nationally promulgated administrative regulations for quality of care review. Such regulations will at the least be directed toward providers serving individuals eligible for direct public programs and other programs planned, initiated, or initially supported by federal grants and loan guarantees. Along with other research provided for in the Health Maintenance Organization Act, this study will accelerate the potential for development of a nationwide pattern of professional review.

The HMO legislation authorizes $50 million over a four year period for studies on definition, measurement, and evaluation of health care quality. The research to be supported must be conducted with attention to both group practice arrangements and fee-for-service solo practice. There is an overriding need for collaborative work between the federal administrators of the HMO and PSRO programs and an accommodation between their apparent differences in degree of aggressiveness toward formulating standard uniform review procedures and practices.

It should be expected that some funds available for research regarding quality measurement will be applied for and contracted to associations representing professions other than medicine. Peer review for physicians is clearly only the beginning. Organized efforts are needed to construct efficient and effective review procedures for all the health professions. The profession next to receive attention in this area is likely to be determined by the relative aggressiveness of various associations in seeking public funds for these purposes. The most likely groups for early involvement would include nursing, podiatry, and pharmacy.

The PSRO law and the quality assurance provision of the HMO bill will shape the environment into which national action will shortly introduce some form of universal health insurance. Any such insurance plan will be accompanied by requirements for relatively stringent resource accounting procedures and for centralized management of presently independent health care institutions and practitioners. The HMO law will expand the experience of government in management of corporations for health care delivery. The PSRO effort will test a control system for cost and quality in three federally financed medical service programs. Experience in these efforts will form the basis for more accurate estimates of economic and social consequences expected under a national health insurance scheme.

The HMO and PSRO efforts do not represent rapid or abrupt innovations in public policy, as both embody concepts and activities with a long history in the United States. They are separate steps in the evolution of public policy and both contribute to the design of a national system for management of an exceedingly vital complex of services similar to systems already in operation in most industrialized countries of the world.

ACKNOWLEDGMENT

I would like to acknowledge the editorial assistance of Mrs. Janet Gelsinger in the preparation of this paper.

REFERENCES

1. Kissick, William L., and Martin, Samuel P.: Issues of the future in health. Annals of the American Academy of Political and Social Science 399:151-159, January 1972.
2. Eilers, Robert D., and Moyerman, Sue S. (eds.): National Health Insurance. Richard D. Irwin, Inc., Homewood, Illinois, 1971.
3. U.S. Congress: Medicare and Medicaid; Problems, Issues, and Alternatives, 91st Congress, first session. U. S. Government Printing Office, Washington, D.C., 1970.
4. Brock, Robert Henry: Quality of Care Assessment: A Comparison of Five Methods of Peer Review. National Center for Health Services Research and Development, U.S. Department of Health, Education and Welfare, Bureau of Health Services Research and Evaluation, July 1973.
5. Donabedian, Avedis: An evaluation of prepaid group practice. Inquiry 6:3-27, September 1969.
6. Donabedian, Avedis: A Review of Some Experiences with Prepaid Group Practice. Research Series No. 12, Bureau of Public Health Economics, University of Michigan School of Public Health, Ann Arbor, Michigan, 1965.
7. Greenlich, Merwyn R.: The impact of prepaid group practice on American medical care: A critical evaluation. Annals of the American Academy of Political and Social Science 399:100-113, January 1972.
8. National Advisory Commission on Health Facilities: A Report to the President. U.S. Government Printing Office, Washington, D.C., 1968.
9. Health Care in America, Part I. Hearings before the Subcommittee on Executive Reorganization of the Committee on Government Operations, U.S. Senate, 90th Congress, 2nd session. U.S. Government Printing Office, Washington, D.C., 1970.
10. Social Policy for Health Care. New York Academy of Medicine, New York, 1969.
11. Kissick, William L. (ed.): Dimensions and determinants of health policy. Milbank Memorial Fund Quarterly, Vol. XLVI, No. 1, Part 2, January 1968.
12. Medical Care for the American People: The Final Report of the Committee on the Costs of Medical Care. University of Chicago Press, Chicago, 1932.
13. Health Maintenance Organization Act of 1973, Public Law 93-222. 93rd Congress, S. 14. U. S. Government Printing Office, Washington D. C., December 29, 1973.

14. Roemer, Milton: A national health system: Analysis and projection. Hospital Progress 50:71-75, Sept. 1969. Reprinted in National Health Insurance, Part 2. Hearings before the Committee on Labor and Public Welfare, U. S. Senate, 91st Congress, 2nd session. U. S. Government Printing Office, Washington, D. C., 1970, pp. 737-745.

15. Somers, H. M., and Somers, A. R.: Critical issues for policy decisions, in Doctors, Patients and Health Insurance. The Brookings Institution, Washington, D. C., 1961.

16. Rosenthal, Gerald: Health care, in The State and the Poor. Cambridge Winthrop Publishers, Inc., 1970, pp. 193-221.

17. Reinhardt, Uwe E.: Proposed changes in the organization of health care delivery: An overview and critique. Milbank Memorial Fund Quarterly, Vol. LI, No. 2, Spring 1973, pp. 193-221.

18. Health Maintenance Organization Act of 1973, op. cit., Part K, Quality Assurance, Section 4, pp. 21-22.

19. Ibid., p. 20.

20. American Medical Association: Peer Review Manual, Vol. 1. Chicago, 1972, Chapter 2, p. 1.

21. American Medical Association: Topics. Chicago, 1972, pp. 130-131.

22. Nichols, Ervin E.: Medicine as seen by Washington in 1973. American Journal of Obstetrics and Gynecology 116:519-530, June 15, 1973.

23. Health Manpower Report, Vol. 2, No. 25, December 11, 1973, p. 5. Capitol Publishers, Inc., Washington, D. C.

24. Social Security Amendments of 1972, Public Law 92-603, 92nd Congress, H.R. 1, Section 249F, p. 102. U. S. Government Printing Office, Washington, D. C., October 30, 1972.

25. Professional standards review: Notice of proposal rule making. Federal Register, Vol. 38, No. 244, Part 2, December 20, 1973.

26. PSROs, here they come—ready or not. Medical World News 14:15-17, March 30, 1973.

27. Health Maintenance Organization Act of 1973, op. cit., Section 1155.

28. Flashner, Bruce A.: U. S. Medicine 9:22, November 15, 1973.

29. U.S. Senate Committee on Finance: Principal Medicare and Medicaid Provisions. Report #92-1230, Section B, pp. 254-269. U. S. Government Printing Office, Washington, D. C., September 26, 1972.

30. Farrell, John R.: PSROs and internal hospital review. Trustee 26:27, November 1973.

Health Policy and the HMO*

ERNEST W. SAWARD, M.D. AND
MERYWYN R. GREENLICK, PH.D.

Policy making is fraught with difficulty. The long-range results are often far afield from the original expectation. This, of course, has been conspicuous in such fields as defense, foreign affairs and economics. Serious attempts to formulate a national policy for the delivery of medical services are relatively new for the United States. Foreseeing the ultimate result of any policy decision is quite difficult. It was certainly not perceived that the laudable Flexner reform of medical education, aided and implemented by the support of medical education through research funds from the federal government, would ultimately create a crisis in the access to primary medical care. The reforming of medical education to change and shorten the medical curriculum, the creation of a "specialty" of primary family practice and the genesis of new health professionals, such as the nurse practitioner and the physician's assistant, are all attempts to ameliorate the effects of a policy decision made sixty years ago. This is not to say that the policy decision was wrong; the inference is that the ultimate results were difficult to foresee.

The past seven years have seen much activity at the federal level in attempts to make health policy. The dominant event is, of course, the modifications of the Social Security Act creating the Medicare and Medicaid programs in 1965. The size of these programs was matched by the size and acrimony of the debate preceding its passage. Parts of the Act creating these programs reflect the thoughts of those who were in advocacy, and indeed, parts of the Act reflect the thoughts of those who were in opposition. It was, in great part, an Act of compromise. Being of very broad scope, many of the provisions were without significant precedent. Many of the decisions about specific items were made with only fragmentary information, for the

*Reprinted from the Milbank Memorial Fund Quarterly, Vol. L, No. 2, Part 1, April 1972, pp. 147-176, with the permission of the authors and the Milbank Memorial Fund.

data were not at hand on which to base policy in a more predictive fashion. The crisis in health care followed quite promptly.

The amendments of the Economic Opportunity Act of 1966 established the authority for the comprehensive Neighborhood Health Center component of the Office of Economic Opportunity. The success or failure of this policy decision over the past five years is not at issue. However, the amount of information available to forecast the results of this innovative series of demonstrations was small indeed, and it is doubtful that what little existed was significantly taken into account in formulating the policies.

The Regional Medical Programs, as envisioned in the DeBakey Committee Report, bear only faint resemblance to the resultant Act (PL 89-239). The Act itself, with its admonishing stricture against changing the organization of the delivery of health services, stands in contrast to the main thrust of the present program, which is, indeed, to change the organization of the delivery of health services. The .Partnership for Health, Comprehensive Health Planning Act (PL 89-749), also displays a significant disparity between the intent of the original health policy and the program practice after a five-year period.

All of these programs, each a major policy decision, each problem-ridden in its execution, were entered upon with high intent but with a very small information base on which to make a decision. There are many more examples. Even a superficial review points up that the data available for decision making are not only scarce but of widely varying quality. This state of affairs leads to assertion, strong advocacy and equally strong denial. Social policy is inevitably based on ideology and not on information. Perhaps this situation is inevitable. Nevertheless, the thought recurs that perhaps more adequate sources of information about health services would lead to the formulation of more accurately predictive policy in this crisis-ridden field.

The size of the stake is huge and is rapidly increasing. The estimates made of the cost of Medicare and Medicaid prior to its implementation in 1966 and the subsequent cost overruns cannot help but remind one of the defense industry. The effect on state budgets of Medicaid has provoked a crisis in local financing and political recriminations that extend far beyond the health field. Some of the remedies advocated, such as institutional price controls and peer review organizations for professionals, would seem to be derived from the homeopathic philosophy.

The nation is at the beginning of a major new thrust in health policy—the era of the Health Maintenance Organization. It has been widely heralded for the past two years. It is one of the policy issues on which the President and his administration, Wilbur Mills and the House Ways and Means Committee, and Senator Kennedy all agree! Although imminent, the Congress has not yet acted on any of the many related proposals.

The name Health Maintenance Organization (HMO) is new in the past two years. Considering the state of the art, it must be considered a politicized euphemism. The vast majority of the work of any such organization that fulfills the requirements being laid down will be sickness care; and, indeed, on the assumption that man is mortal, it will probably remain so into the future. However, with that caveat, the HMO is intended to provide the inherent motivation for any prevention and any cost-effective disease detection that exists.

Inasmuch as the term Health Maintenance Organization is not self-revealing as to the concepts implied, it is necessary to make them more explicit. The noun in the term Health Maintenance Organization is "organization," and the first provision is that there be an organization of comprehensive medical services with the understanding of a guaranteed access to these services in relation to medical need. The second provision is that of an enrolled population that has had a choice of systems of medical care and has voluntarily chosen the HMO.

Finally, the costs of all care are to be mutualized among the defined population so that a total budget is funded. The budget is then paid by contract to the providers of care, both professional and institutional, who, in turn, agree to deliver their respective services for an agreed-upon-in-advance capitation. The resultant dynamic is to convert morbidity from its usual status as an asset of the providers to the status of a liability to them. Hence, the provider, like the consumer, has his economic interest in morbidity prevention. Thereby the rather optimistic name of Health Maintenance Organization.

The President, in his health message of November 18, 1971, states:[1]

In recent years, a new method for delivering health services has achieved growing respect. This new approach has two essential attributes. It brings together a comprehensive range of medical services in a single organization so that a patient is assured of convenient access to all of them. And it provides needed services for a fixed-contract fee which is paid in advance by all subscribers.

Such an organization can have a variety of forms and names and sponsors. One of the strengths of this new concept, in fact, is its great flexibility. The general term which has been applied to all of these units is HMO—Health Maintenance Organization.

The most important advantage of Health Maintenance Organizations is that they increase the value of the services a consumer receives for each health dollar. This happens first because such organizations provide a strong financial incentive for better preventive care and for greater efficiency.

Under traditional systems, doctors and hospitals are paid, in effect, on a piecework basis. The more illnesses they treat—and the more service they render— the more their income rises.

This does not mean, of course, that they do any less than their very best to make people well. But it does mean that there is no economic incentive for them to concentrate on keeping people healthy.

A fixed-price contract for comprehensive care reverses this illogical incentive. Under this arrangement, income grows not with the number of days a person is sick but with the number of days he is well. HMO's therefore have a strong fi-

nancial interest in preventing illness, or, failing that, in treating it in its early-
stages, promoting a thorough recovery and preventing any reoccurrence. Like
doctors in ancient China, they are paid to keep their clients healthy. For them,
economic interests work to reinforce their professional interests.

And the House Committee on Ways and Means in its report to the Congress states:[2]

Your committee believes that a serious problem in the present approach to
payment for services in the health field, either by private patients, private insurance or the government, is that, in effect, payment is made to the provider
for each individual service performed, so that other things being equal, there is
an economic incentive on the part of those who make the decisions on what
services are needed to provide more services, services that may not be essential
and even unnecessary services.

A second major problem is that, ordinarily, the individual must largely find his
own way among various types and levels of services with only partial help from
a single hospital, a nursing home, a home health agency, various specialists
and so on. No one takes responsibility, in a large proportion of the cases, for
determining the appropriate level of care in total and for seeing that such care,
but no more, is supplied.

The pattern of operation of Health Maintenance Organizations that provide
services on a per capita prepayment basis lends itself to a solution of both these
problems with respect to the care of individuals enrolled with them. Because
the organization receives a fixed annual payment from enrollees regardless of
the volume of services rendered, there is a financial incentive to control costs
and to provide only the least expensive service that is appropriate and adequate
for the enrollee's needs. Moreover, such organizations take responsibility for
deciding which services the patient should receive and then seeing that those
are the services he gets.

Secretary Elliot Richardson, in the White Paper of May, 1971, after
reiterating in similar words the idea and motivation of HMO's, describes the findings that interest the government in this form of organization.[3]

In contrast with more traditional and alternative modes of care, HMO's show
lower utilization rates for the most expensive types of care (measured by hospital days in particular); they tend to reduce the consumer's total health-care
outlay; and—the ultimate test—they appear to deliver services of high quality.
Available research studies show that HMO members are more likely than
other population groups to receive such preventive measures as general
checkups and prenatal care, and to seek care within one day of the onset of
symptoms of illness or injuries.

The sources cited for these conclusions are from the studies of Denson, et al., and Shapiro, et al., and from the Social Security Administration, Office of Research and Statistics on the Medicare Program.

In his remarks before the American Hospital Association in Chicago on August 24, 1971, the Secretary stated: "I am firmly convinced that at this time, no alternatives are superior to ours in the strength of their base of knowledge . . . ."[4] The Secretary, however, clearly pointed out the state of the art in this manner:[5]

> I should like to say, however, in passing, that our proposals evolved out of an examination of literally hundreds of options. And one of our judgmental criteria was: how far may we go with an option given our state of knowledge.
>
> In some instances, we found the knowledge to be extensive, sufficiently so to propose sweeping changes. In other instances, we were brought up sharply by the taut reins of ignorance. We were wary then, and are wary now, of panaceas calling for universal and abrupt changes, where the base of knowledge is so fragile it can support little more than fancy.

The American Medical Association is, however, unconvinced. In its publication on Health Maintenance Organizations of May, 1971, quoting its testimony before the Senate finance Committee on H.R. 17550, the Association states:[6]

> We believe that cost and utilization data should first be developed with control demonstrations testing the capability of such a program to accomplish its purpose. There are questions regarding in-fact cost savings, as well as the quality of health care which may be provided when there are economic incentives to providers to reduce utilization.

These statements, that of Secretary Richardson as to no alternatives being superior in regard to the strength of the base of knowledge, and the American Medical Association's forthright skepticism, rather well stake out the ground of debate on the validity of the HMO strategy. Many secondary grounds of debate concern financing, tactics of promotion, what manner of organizations might qualify and many other derivative issues, but all pend on the nature of evidence that the HMO is, indeed, a better way.

As previously mentioned, the name Health Maintenance Organization in its present connotation is new in the past two years. However, the notions that lie behind the name are not new. It is always hard to say when ideas originate, and, in fact, they often keep being reinvented. The President, in his health message, cited the idea's being present in ancient China, and inasmuch as this has been oft cited over the years, there may be some substance to it. A Chinese scholar, however, and one professionally engaged in working with these concepts, has stated that he has had great difficulty authenticating any widespread use of the notion in ancient

China.[7] Medical mutuals and "Friendly Societies" with similar ideas did indeed exist in the nineteenth century in Europe and the lands that had been colonized by Europeans.

The most significant, reasoned and detailed approach in the United States stems from the series of reports of the Committee on the Cost of Medical Care, reporting from 1927 to 1932, that advocated prepayment and group practice as specific policies for rationalizing the American medical care system.[8] The professional founder of the Kaiser Foundation Medical Care Program, which dates back to 1933, has reported that he was not influenced by this report, inasmuch as it did not come to his attention until many years after the program he founded was already successful.[9] Perhaps this offers a lesson for those who spend considerable portions of their time sitting on committees studying health policy. Theoretical hypotheses are often of little avail without viable examples.

Most of the prototype organizations that now would qualify as HMO's had their origins in the 1930's and 1940's, and most of the evidence in regard to cost and utilization comes from those organizations. They have been known as prepaid group practices. Each was involved in controversy from its origin. Organized medicine, which would now like to develop controlled demonstrations, originally was restrained from annihilating them only by federal and state Supreme Court decisions. The American Medical Association arrived at an alleged neutral position with the Larson Committee Report of 1959.[10] Many of the constituent medical societies, however, have taken much longer to arrive at such a neutral position, if indeed they have.

None of this long debate appeared to influence the federal government in arriving at a Health Maintenance Organization policy. It was only with medical care cost escalation and the resultant budgetary dilemmas, particularly as they affected the Medicare and Medicaid programs, that the executive and legislative branches of the government became sensitized and aware of any options.

The Medicare law, as passed in 1965, mentioned prepaid group practice and capitation payment as a result of the prepaid group practice organizations' efforts to modify the law to allow their usual manner of program function. However, to this day, and despite several modifications of the law, the prepaid group practice programs remain functioning on a cost reimbursement basis, a process quite at variance with prospective budgeting.

The attempts, however, to make the Social Security Administration and the Congress aware of these difficulties and the resultant data comparing the health care utilization of the elderly under these programs with the national averages proved to be a very salutary exercise. It is largely on the basis of these data and the data flowing from the Federal Employees Health Benefits Act of 1959 that the federal government became aware of its option. Reports of various study groups and commissions have underlined these differences,[11] but if it were not for the involvement of the Congress with the funding of its own creations, sensitivities to such reports would be markedly less.

As these data developed year after year, together with conceptual arguments to elucidate why such data resulted from these programs,[12] government authorities became progressively more interested. When, finally, in July of 1969, the President proclaimed a health crisis and called for significant innovation in the health care system, the examination of options became inevitable. The approach of the prepaid group practices was clearly being advocated as the solution to the American health care crisis. What was the information on hand at that time concerning prepaid group practices on which sufficient judgments about HMO's could be made? What was the quality of the data? What information might have been available, considering the state of the art, and in what way might the state of the art be advanced in a practical manner to significantly contribute to policy making? Examining the state of the art relative to social policy concerning the HMO is instructive in assessing data needs in health policy generally. Certainly many of the questions are the same and many of the data are equally available.

Evaluating the effectiveness of a medical care form, such as prepaid group practice, requires the measuring of that form's performance against its stated goals.[13] In medical care the goals are to reduce morbidity, minimize disability and avoid premature death. Measuring effectiveness has two components. The first is the measurement of the technical performance of the system. The second assessment relates to measuring the form's acceptance; how well, for example, prepaid group practice has gained acceptance by the population and by the providers of care. Unfortunately, research in each of these areas has been limited, and it has been difficult to draw any definitive conclusions.

Donabedian indicates that the evaluation of quality can proceed by evaluating the structure, process and outcome of the medical care system.[14] It is possible to use this framework in the assessment of effectiveness of prepaid group practice. This type of evaluation does not answer specific questions about the health of the populations of prepaid group practice programs. Rather, it asserts that when an appropriate structure and an appropriate process are developed and certain outcomes can be observed, these outcomes will affect positively the health of the population. This approach seems reasonable, but the ultimate evaluation, of course, must determine if belonging to a prepaid group practice program improves the health status of the population enrolled. Little evidence exists that personal health services provided in any current system materially affect the health status of populations. The scientific problems of measurement and the difficulties of experimental design in medical care are constraints.

We are left with the assessment of structure, process and a limited outcome in evaluating prepaid group practice relative to the remaining medical care systems. For example, it has been argued that integrating care in a hospital-based system, providing the centralization inherent in the use of a single medical record and making available all needed resources under central administrative control provide the potential for making appropriate services available at all times. If there are no financial barriers to care and if all appropriate services are available, an increased probability exists that care will be of adequate quality.

Further, it is argued that the medical care system can be organized to minimize the motivation for physicians to proceed inappropriately. It can avoid, for example, providing financial incentives to unnecessarily hospitalize patients or to perform unnecessary surgery. In prepaid group practice the relation between the financing system and the organization of medical care is critical in structuring the environment to avoid motivation for such undesirable behavior. The capitation payment to physicians, by providing the group a fixed income for each person enrolled in the system, is designed to facilitate use of appropriate service.

It has been asserted that in prepaid group practice the colleague interaction is an important determinant of quality, even though little experimental evidence exists concerning this point. Such factors as the ready availability of all specialties, the ease of consultation and the easy exchange of information can be viewed as positively influencing the quality of care. On the other hand, it has been argued that social pressure can be applied for inappropriate behavior as well as appropriate behavior in an organized situation. In the highly structured situation of group practice organizations, attitudes, good or bad, concerning quality and appropriate utilization of services will be reflected in the practice pattern of physicians.

In a tightly knit prepaid group practice structure, it is simple to institute peer review on the behavior of individual physicians. The providers of care have to use and see each other's work because of the unit medical record. It is assummed that this unit record leads to better quality. In the unorganized system, records are maintained by one man and are not subject to the critical review of general use, except in the hospital. The contemporary demand for peer review has caused county medical societies throughout the country to attempt to develop peer review mechanisms in the solo practice, fee-for-service system.

Differential outcomes resulting from the process and structural differences in prepaid group practice systems appear as utilization pattern differences. In particular, there is reduction in surgery on patients of prepaid group practice physicians and some increases in the use of preventive services. Donabedian, for example, has concluded that tentative evidence indicates that unjustified surgery tends to be less frequent in a prepaid group practice program.[15] He refers particularly to the much lower tonsillectomy rates in prepaid group practice in the federal employees health benefit program. He cites differences in overall hospitalization rates and in rates for surgical procedures among group practice patients. He further cites data indicating that preventive services are used more frequently by members of prepaid group practice programs, particularly higher utilization for cervical cytology examination and more appropriate use of general and prenatal checkups among members of the group practice plans. A higher proportion of group practice members make contact with a physician each year, thereby increasing the probability of preventive care. Data are limited in these areas, however, both with regard to behavior within the prepaid group practice program and to data deriving from the solo practice, fee-for-service system.

As has been mentioned many times, most Kaiser physicians are either board certified or board eligible and the system's hospitals are all approved by the Joint Commission for the Accreditation of Hospitals. This is true to a varying degree in other group practices. These are structural features generally considered to be related to quality. Also, Kaiser, HIP and increasingly other prepaid group practice plans have research units that continually assess various aspects of system performance and feed results back into the system. Such systematic research is rarely attempted in other segments of the medical care system because neither a defined population base nor an integrated unit record system are available. This type of research provides at least the potential for assessing and therefore affecting quality.

In evaluating the effectiveness of the prepaid group practice organizations, assessment of the acceptance factors is certainly indicated. How does participation in this system affect satisfaction with medical care by both the patients and the providers of care? Evidence on consumer and professional satisfaction is fairly scanty, although work has proceeded since Friedson's classic work.[16] It is possible, however, to make two broad generalizations about this question of consumer satisfaction. First, the great majority in any medical care system appear to be fairly well satisfied with the health services they have. In addition, there appears to be a hard core of the dissatisfied, perhaps as high as ten per cent, who dislike many things about the medical care system in which they participate.[17]

The major problem in evaluating consumer satisfaction with prepaid group practice programs is the difficulty of answering the question: Compared to what? Significant dissatisfaction with the arrangements of medical care is being expressed throughout the United States. Significant numbers have no arrangements. Various consumer-oriented groups have been attacking much of the medical care system, but, particularly, they have been raising questions concerned with participant satisfaction.

The statement has been made that members of the Kaiser Foundation Medical Care Program are generally satisfied with their medical care system. The system serves more than two million members, having had a very high growth rate. The dual or multiple choice requirement of the Kaiser Program indicates this growth is based on periodic individual decisions and not on majority action of groups. On the other hand, prepaid group practice programs have not attained this high growth rate in some parts of the country.

A survey recently completed on a sample of the Kaiser membership in Portland indicates significant general satisfaction with the medical care system, but also indicates the pervasiveness of certain typical criticisms.[18] A large proportion of people interviewed recalled they joined Kaiser because of recommendations from friends or relatives. Generally the participants' motivation for joining Kaiser was financial rather than a view that the organization of care was significantly better than care in the community in general. These data may indicate that the total coverage of services at a reasonable premium is the prime attraction of the system. After receiving service in the system, the members appeared relatively satisfied with the quality of care, the cost, the facilities and the physician characteristics generally, but appear to express some dissatisfaction with particular system characteristics, including waiting time for an appointment. Less than six per cent suggested that Kaiser physicians were not as good as physicians outside of Kaiser, whereas nearly twenty per cent felt they were better. The majority said they were about the same.

The above data are generally consistent with Donabedian's conclusions that the majority of subscribers to group practice plans are satisfied with their plan in spite of the substantial differences in the various plans. He points out that the subscribers who complain about medical care have a great many things about which to complain. He states that an appreciable proportion of complaints made by subscribers of prepaid group practice plans are applicable to medical care generally.[19]

The existence of an organized system provides the capability of changing the factors causing unhappiness among consumers of care. The Group Health Cooperative in Seattle, for example, is controlled by an active consumer board that is greatly concerned with matters of consumer satisfaction. The role of the consumer in the development of this prepaid group practice program has been well detailed by MacColl.[20]

The basic belief in the consumer's right to purchase his preference has been put forth as important in controlling provider behavior. However, because the supply of medical care practitioners is relatively tight, the right to withhold his dollar from the providers of services if dissatisfied is a very weak control. The potential exists for organized consumer groups to influence the behavior of the medical care system and to increase satisfaction within the system. This is one of the goals of health maintenance organization development. The federal legislation pending is likely to have mandates for consumer involvement in the planning and provision of services in HMO's.[21] Consumer control has been more or less implemented in the Office of Economic Opportunity (OEO) Neighborhood Health Center projects, but the score has not yet been tallied on the relation between consumer satisfaction and the degree of consumer influence and control in the system. It is possible that the level of patient satisfaction is no different in organizations controlled by consumers than in organizations controlled by the suppliers of care.

Data are almost nonexistent concerning the satisfaction of physicians in prepaid group practice, and it is nonexistent concerning the relative satisfaction of the other personnel in the system. Some feel that, in general, physicians participating in prepaid group practices are satisfied with this type of arrangement. Conceptually, at least, group practice is designed to increase physician satisfaction. The freedom from concern with the mundane business operations of medical practice, the ability to arrange hours and to limit the excessive burdens of long night and weekend calls, the ready availability of various fringe benefits and the easy access and social support of working with a group of esteemed colleagues combine to make group practice an apparently favorable work environment. Whereas the reports from medical directors of prepaid group practice organizations in the 1950's and early 1960's reflected the difficulties of recruiting adequate physicians,[22] recent reports indicate recruiting is only difficult because of the present inadequate supply of physicians in certain specialty fields of practice. Recruitment of physicians for prepaid group practice programs has become relatively successful.

Published data, again from the Kaiser-Permanente medical care system, indicate a low turnover rate for physicians once they become involved with the program. The Kaiser medical care system is organized by contracting for medical services with autonomous partnerships of physicians, the various Permanente Medical Groups. The partnerships hire new physicians as salaried employees for periods from two to three years. At the end of this probationary period, acceptable physicians are taken into the partnership. Data for the years 1966 through 1970 from the Permanente Medical Group indicate an average turnover rate of less than ten per cent per year for employed physicians in the probationary period and less than two per cent per year for the partners.[23]

A recent study published by Smith is one of the few to even explore the attitudes of other personnel in prepaid group practice programs.[24] This study does not provide the basis for comparison, but there is little reason to believe that personnel would be any less satisfied working in hospitals or ambulatory care facilities associated with prepaid group practice programs. Certainly the availability of pension and other benefits and the stability of working in a large organization might increase satisfaction for most.

In general, much work remains to be done in assessing acceptance factors. Particular attention should be paid to the concomitant relation between satisfaction and the behavior of patients and providers within the system. It might be possible to evaluate the acceptance factors of prepaid group practice programs and other medical care systems, differentiating those factors that relate to the financing of the system from those that relate to the organization of care.

Much of the social policy discussion concerning the HMO is brought about because of asserted economic advantages of the prepaid group practice arrangements. These arguments can only be assessed in light of the evaluation of the efficiency of this form of organization. In a review of economic research in group medicine, Klarman points out that the expected savings from group practice medicine might include two major components: economies of scale in the production of services and a lower rate of hospital utilization widely associated with the prepaid form of group practice.[25] However, to adequately evaluate the efficiences of prepaid group practice, it is necessary to assess the total input needed to produce required services for a population of given characteristics. Prepaid group practice should be viewed as a medical care delivery system that accepts responsibility for the organization, financing and delivery of health care services to a defined population. The attainment of this definition ought to set the bounds for this evaluation.

There is little reason to believe that the contributions of prepaid group practice in the efficiency of medical care would be from efficiencies of scale. Efficiencies of scale, deriving from internal operating efficiencies of a medical care organization, ought not be expected to provide a significant magnitude of savings even if they do exist. For example, there is no reason to believe that a prepaid group practice system could produce a single unit of hospital care more economically than another hospital of the same size. Nor is there even reason to believe that the prepaid group practice system could produce any single doctor office visit more cheaply than other practitioners.

Nevertheless, the expenditures for producing medical care services for a total population covered by prepaid group practice programs are less than the expenditures for care to similar populations covered in the traditional solo fee-for-service system. These expenditure differences arise from what can properly be called the "system efficiencies" of prepaid group practice. The reductions in expenditure for the care of total populations derive from many sources. It is clear that the populations covered by prepaid group practice programs use fewer days of hospital care per person in the population than do similar populations in the community system, even when utilization outside of the system is taken into account.

The organization of the total medical care system, including financing factors, medical practice factors, facility supply factors, all act in the same direction to maintain the lower use of hospitals by the total population. By integrating fiscal responsibility with the organization of medical care, prepaid group practice can reduce incentives for the physician or the population to prefer that inappropriate services be provided on an inpatient basis. Services in or out of hospital are financed in the same manner. The full range of services can be made available within a prepaid group practice program, so that physicians and population find inpatient, ambulatory care, diagnostic and most other services equally available.

The impact of these phenomena can be seen in historical data from Kaiser, Portland.[26] As the cost per day of hospitalization rose in the Kaiser Hospital in Portland from $13.23 per patient day in 1950 to $54.80 per day in 1966, paralleling the national increase, the cost of hospitalization per member year increased from $12.53 in 1950 to $27.31 in 1966. A four-fold increase per patient day was reflected as a two-fold plus increase in cost per member per year because the use of hospital days per person per year in the population decreased concurrently. It is this difference in the rate of increase in cost per day and cost per person per year that accounts for the difference in the cost of hospitalization for the Kaiser-Portland population relative to the remainder of the community.

A similar perspective must be taken to evaluate the potential of prepaid group practice programs for appropriate use of manpower in the United States. Bailey questions the relative efficiency of group practice in the production of medical services by relating the number of ancillary personnel per physician and the number of visits per physician in various sizes of group practice.[27] However, the more relevant measure, and the one that really defines the impact of the system efficiencies, is the number of physicians and other personnel required to provide the total medical care services for a population.

Stevens has estimated the number of physicians that would be needed to provide medical care to the American population, other things being equal, if the relative ratio of physicians to population for the United States totally was equal to that of Kaiser-Portland.[28] He estimates the need to be ten per cent fewer physicians than were, in fact, available in the United States.

These data were not meant to imply that it would have been possible to provide care for the total population of the country in a Kaiser-like system, but rather to point out the possibility of other solutions to the problem of the current disequilibrium in physician services other than simply increasing the number of physicians. The study is cited here to point out the difference between Bailey's approach of evaluating efficiency by looking at efficiencies of scale and Stevens' approach of assessing "system efficiencies." Stevens asks, "What are the inputs necessary to provide service to the entire population?" and not, "What are the inputs necessary to produce a given unit of service?"

Data are now available that bear on the magnitude of outside utilization in Kaiser, and particularly in Kaiser in Portland. The above-mentioned survey of members of the Health Plan in Portland gathered information on the outside utilization of members. Preliminary tabulations of these data indicate that about ten per cent of the population had at least one use of outside medical care services in the twelve months preceding the interview. A characteristic use was for the member new to the system to use his old source of service for a minor problem. These services accounted for considerably less than ten per cent of the total services used by the population, and a significant portion was for services paid for by and known to the medical care system.

Critics have asserted that the use of hospitalization in prepaid group practice programs represents an underutilization of hospital services. Considering that the technology has not yet been developed to appropriately measure differences in health status in populations, it can only be said that the population using medical care services in prepaid group practices with a hospital base of two beds per 1,000 does not appear to be any less healthy or appear to have any higher mortality rates, than do populations receiving hospital care in a system utilizing four hospital beds per 1,000. In contradiction to more equating with better, one must be cognizant of the risk of iatrogenic, hospital-based disease.

It is quite clear that two different forms of organization are envisaged in the Health Maintenance Organization concept. Prepaid group practice is obviously the dominant idea, and the data derived to support the HMO have been derived from prepaid group practice, as seen in the Secretary's White Paper.[29] Further, in speaking of the HMO concept, the President has referred to "one-stop shopping" as part of it. Obviously, "one-stop shopping" in regard to the HMO can only mean the centralized, integrated, organized group practice model.

However, another model is extant—the medical foundation, or decentralized model, in which services are rendered in each individual physician's office. The medical foundation model quite clearly stems from experience of the San Joaquin Medical Foundation. This program, founded by the San Joaquin Medical Society under the leadership of Dr. Donald Harrington, dates from 1954. Part of the impetus for its creation stems indirectly from prepaid group practice. The International Longshoremen's and Warehousemen's Union on the Pacific Coast had initiated a coastwise contract for prepaid group practice for its members who lived in areas where prepaid group practice was available (the major West Coast ports) with service starting in January, 1950.

After a few years' experience the Union was more satisfied with the medical care provided in those areas that had prepaid group practice. In response to the Kaiser Program's being urged by the Union to extend its services to the inland Sacramento River ports in 1954, the San Joaquin Medical Society arranged the prototype of the present foundation program with representatives of this union and the employer association. The program was then extended to other groups who wished to enroll. An insurance carrier served as the intermediary, setting the premium rates and underwriting the liability.

The principles of the foundation methodology, as they evolved, included an insistence upon broad, comprehensive coverage, so that the appropriate services could be used; a fixed fee schedule acceptable to all participating physicians as full payment; and peer review of the medical performance of the collaborating physicians so that quality could be reviewed. Quality, in this context, was defined as appropriateness of the medical care process for the presumed diagnosis. Claims for services that were judged inappropriate were to be denied.

The medical foundation concept at this stage of development lacked one of the elements considered essential to the HMO concept. It had no prospective budget or capitation in which the providers are put at risk for the responsibility for the delivery of comprehensive services. There has been an experiment with this approach for "MediCal" in the past two years, with asserted cost savings to that program. On the basis of this limited operational experience as underwriters, the medical foundations have become the decentralized model of HMO. The active role of advocacy of the HMO option by the medical foundations has gained wide Congressional support.

One of the repeated statements of the administration is that there are to be possible many innovative forms of HMO. Almost every form put forward so far has been a variant of the prepaid group practice or medical foundation model, with some that seem to be combinations of the two. No totally new idea has come forward. It should be emphasized that neither prepaid group practice nor the medical foundation is a monolithic concept,[30] there being a wide range of varieties of each.

Countervailing forces are at work in the federal government in sponsorship of the HMO option. Foremost, perhaps, is the urgency to implement such a program so that this choice will be available to a significant portion of the American public in a significant number of places in this decade. This is a monumental task, and some of the difficulties have been detailed elsewhere.[31] The opposing tendency on the part of the government is to make rules and regulations sufficiently constraining so that this new system cannot be abused. The potential for abuse is significant. The abuses that have occurred within the Medicare and Medicaid programs have been well publicized, and the administrators of these programs have felt the heat of Congressional investigation. They are naturally inclined to protect themselves by creating rules and regulations that would provide meaningful control to prevent such abuse. H.R. 11728, the Health Maintenance Act of 1971, submitted by Congressman William Roy of Kansas, is quite precise in defining an HMO.[32]

The paradox, of course, is that the professional providers of health service outside of HMO's find themselves under very little control and constrained by very few rules and regulations. In general, there is an open-ended payment system, where each piece of work performed has a "usual and customary" price tag, and the manner of enterprise is quite free indeed. The only constraint is against fraud. The providers are being asked to take advantage of the health maintenance option under detailed constraints. They are being asked to underwrite the risk financially within a prospective budget, with which most have had very little experience. Although interest is high in the HMO concept, it should not be expected that this phenomenon, like Asian flu, will sweep the country within a few months.

The public may be strongly motivated to want this type of access to organized services on a budgeted basis. But what of the incentives to the provider, particularly the professional provider, who at present has very few constraints, in either the way he practices or the way he is rewarded? Marginal economic incentives, depending on his underwriting risk, may be enough to arouse his curiosity and even enough to move professionals to apply for planning grants for HMO's. But when the totality of constraints and their implication become clear, the enthusiasm for operations may diminish.

Certainly, to many in the profession the decentralized model of HMO, the medical foundation, seems a much less radical transformation of their present way of practice. However, a hard look at past experiences in this realm is not encouraging. The Medical Service Bureaus in the Pacific Northwest were prototype HMO's created in response to the depressed financial circumstances of the 1930's. Underwriting commonly resulted in the payment of a pro rata reduction of the nominal fee schedule. This made for unhappy physicians. The physician tended to distinguish the patients who paid him a full fee from those who returned to him a pro rata reduction or discounted fee. Characteristically the latter fee was distinguished as a second-class fee, and, hence, the patient became, pari passu, a second-class patient. This made for unhappy patients as well as unhappy physicians. Although these early models were not exact prototypes of the present day HMO, their operational similarity was close enough to be a warning as to the generalization of this phenomenon.

It has been often asserted that these medical care systems cater essentially to the working populations; that the socioeconomic population distribution is truncated because the very poor and the wealthy are not included. Particularly if poor populations are excluded, HMO's are not likely to have widespread significance in solving the problems in universal access to medical care.

Population groups covered by most group practice programs in the United States were enrolled through occupational groups. Since 1950, health care entitlement has usually been a fringe benefit of employment. The early history of most of the prepaid group practices in existence is dominated by the enrollment of large groups that formed the nucleus for the growth of that program. HIP was stimulated almost entirely by enrollment of city employees in New York. The Kaiser Foundation Health Plan of Oregon was dominated early by its relation with the longshoremen's union; Community Health Association in Detroit by the United Auto Workers, and the Group Health Association of Washington, D. C., by the federal employees.

Although most of the prepaid group practice programs have diversified their memberships and now provide service to members of all of the socioeconomic classes, the distribution of members is not yet equivalent to the general community distribution. Those without entitlement by employment are underrepresented. This, of course, is true of all health insurance in this country.

The prepaid group practice programs gained experience in dealing with federal funding agencies because of Medicare. A significant proportion of the membership of various programs was over 65 years of age, and it was necessary to develop a modus operandi for collecting governmental payments for the provision of services. The process was initially difficult, as previously mentioned, because the federal government could not deal with capitation payments.[33]

When the amendments to the Economic Opportunity Act were passed in 1966, establishing authority for the Neighborhood Health Center component of OEO, two prepaid group practice programs, the Medical Foundation of Bellaire, Ohio,[34] and Kaiser, Portland,[35] were funded as OEO Neighborhood Health Centers. These group practice programs offered the poor an opportunity to participate in established medical care systems already delivering health services to a diverse group in the same geographic area.

This approach was significant because it obviated the time, expense and complexity of building, staffing and organizing new and segregated medical care facilities for the poverty group. The group practice organizations indicated that facilities already existed in many poor areas that could be utilized for the provision of health care services for the indigent. These programs demonstrated the feasibility of organizing and delivering health care through existing medical care systems, although it was necessary to finance care from the public sector.

The two programs appeared to succeed in their objectives,[36] and other prepaid group practice programs have developed ways to provide medical care to poverty groups, including the Group Health Cooperative of Seattle, the Kaiser Foundation of Southern California and Hawaii, the Group Health Association of Washington, D. C., the Community Health Association of Detroit, the Harvard Community Health Foundation, and HIP. There is little reason to believe that the prepaid group practice programs cannot accept a proportionate share of the indigent population into their system. What appear necessary are financing mechanisms that are flexible enough to deal with the capitation form of payment and stable enough to produce continuity of membership.

A genuine concern of the medical foundation type of HMO is its ability to deliver health services to the urban poor. The centralized prepaid group practice model of the HMO quite clearly can create a Neighborhood Health Center and organize services to be delivered to whatever population lives in proximity, and this has been demonstrated, although on a limited scale because of the inability to obtain the financing for a massive test.[37] The problem with the decentralized foundation model is that the individual physicians have largely left the ghetto area in which the urban poor reside, and therefore physical access to the physicians, who are in numbers in suburbia, has little practicality for this population.

For HMO's in general the critical deficit of the poor is their lack of effective entitlement. The nature of Medicaid financing, creating large local tax burdens, constrains the program from implementing the original intent of Title 19. If the costs of the population to be served in an HMO must be mutualized on an equitable basis and the Title 19 mechanism is inadequate, the disadvantaged will be excluded. Only by falling back upon the much larger base of direct federal revenues can the poor effectively participate in HMO programs.

For an HMO to function on a forecast budget and make comprehensive services available on a continuous basis to those who recognize themselves as members of such a program, there cannot be any "on-again-off-again" eligibility status. Eligibility and membership must be on the same basis as most negotiated groups and the federal employees, with the opportunity for enrollment and disenrollment being usually no greater than annual. The difficulties cited, which are formidable, stand in the way, at this time, of general implementation of the HMO option for the impoverished, either in the form of prepaid group practice or in the form of medical foundations, unless there is, by legislation, new federal entitlement.

These options, therefore, are not completely feasible without a form of national health insurance that provides adequate financing for comprehensive medical care and provides it in such a way that eligibility is continuous and without categorization. Furthermore, the incentives for HMO's, at present, in view of the simultaneous constraints as cited above, are not so great as to produce significant change. A form of national health insurance that truly provides equal sums of monies for equal numbers of people of the same characteristics may lead to a reasonably rapid reorganization of the delivery of health services. But to expect one group of providers to accept risk, regulation and a closed-end financial system while leaving others in an unregulated, open-ended system is unreasonable.

It is interesting to contemplate the special dilemma of the medical schools and their interest in the HMO option.[38] In summary, the schools are seriously underfunded. They are dissatisfied with their organization of ambulatory care and ambulatory care teaching. On initial study of these factors, the HMO option appears as a solution to both problems. However, most schools, by tradition and location, are involved with indigent populations with inadequate entitlement. Furthermore, there is inherently little faculty dedication to the responsibilities of continuous primary care. If an HMO is to be voluntary as to membership and self-sustaining as to premiums, how are the teaching costs to be paid, in view of the competitive nature of the option? These issues have been explored elsewhere.[39]

It is clear that we need to know much more about how all HMO's operate, particularly from the consumer viewpoint. Much of the information could be gathered from the presently operating examples. Federal funding for this practical research has not been forthcoming. No agency seems to feel primarily responsible for funding such studies. But when this is accomplished in depth across large samples of the various delivery systems, policy making will be on a firmer base.

The HMO policy is thus a rather classic example of federal policy making in health. Considerable reliance is being placed on this alternate form of health services delivery system to contain the costs of health care. But the likelihood of widespread successful implementation under present circumstances is doubtful. This is not because the HMO does not have merit, but because the present fee-for-service pattern is left with most of the rewards and few of the constraints.

The total national expenditures on health care from all sources for the federal fiscal year 1974 are officially forecast at $105,400,000,000, if no new legislation is enacted.[40] All proposed new legislation increases this huge total. This is one dollar of each thirteen in the projected GNP. More people will be involved in "providing health" than in growing food. Despite the size and scope of this expenditure, it is not uncommon for physicians to express the wish that medical care were not such a political issue! It is evident that any activity taking one dollar in thirteen will remain in the forefront of political action regardless of the kind of legislation passed or not passed. An analogy may be made with agriculture. Ever since the Secretary, Henry Wallace, asked that the little pigs be destroyed, there has never ceased to be a controversy about the farm policy in Congress and in the nation, and never has a policy been produced that pleased all. Because of its size and its personal significance, "health care" will repeat this process with even greater intensity and acrimony.

Medical care research, under these circumstances, must inevitably grow and develop new sophistication and productivity. If the product of the medical care process is to be better health, then health must be defined in a way that can be better measured. A generally accepted yardstick or index of this state would be a significant advance. Measuring the outcome in terms of health by examining various medical care processes has been extraordinarily difficult. Counting the pieces of the process, the dollars, the manpower, the days of hospitalization, the office visits, the technical tests performed and so forth, has been an inadequate substitute for outcome measurement, but unfortunately reflects the state of the art.

The National Center for Health Services Research and Development, an agency of the Department of Health, Education, and Welfare, was created in 1967 to serve the nation in the function its name implies. It is apparently not a field in which quick results are to be expected. Edgar Trevor Williams, the Secretary of the Rhodes Trust of Oxford, in a speech[41] at Chicago, reviewed the role the Nuffield Foundation had played in the United Kingdom in relation to the National Health Service. It had been the sponsor of research, and then demonstration, on a scale just large enough to be significant, testing the interjection of new ideas and processes into the National Health Service. The result often so clarified an issue that it led the bureaucracy into implementing the reform on full national scale. Our National Center has not yet played this role, if this is even an expected part of its mission.

It may remain for private funds to undertake this risk-laden role. It is probably much more than coincidence that the current presidents of some of the major American foundations have been drawn from the physician leaders of medical care administration. It may be that with their support of health care research, health policy can be made from a much more secure information base in the future.

REFERENCES

1.   United States Congress, 92nd Congress: Health message from President of the United States relative to building national health strategy. House Document No. 49, February 18, 1971.
2.   United States Congress, House Committee on Ways and Means: Social Security Amendments of 1971; Report on H.R. 1. House Report No. 92-231, 92nd Congress, 1st Session, 1971, p. 89.
3.   United States Department of Health, Education, and Welfare: Towards a

Comprehensive Health Policy for the 1970s, A White Paper. U. S. Government Printing Office, Washington, D.C., May 1971, p. 32.

4. Richardson, E. L.: Remarks before the American Hospital Association. Chicago, August 24, 1971, p. 2 (mimeograph copy).

5. Ibid., pp. 1, 2.

6. American Medical Association, Division of Medical Practice: HMO's as Seen by the AMA: An Analysis. May, 1971, p. 6.

7. Chu, P.: Personal communication.

8. Committee on the Costs of Medical Care: Medical Care for the American People; Final Report, adopted October 31, 1932. University of Chicago Press, Chicago, 1932. Reprinted by the U. S. Department of Health, Education, and Welfare, Public Health Service, Health Services and Mental Health Administration, Community Health Service, 1970.

9. Garfield, S. R.: Personal communication.

10. Larson, Leonard, W., et al.: Report of the Commission on Medical Care. J.A.M.A., Special Edition, January 17, 1959.

11. National Advisory Commission on Health Manpower: Report. U. S. Government Printing Office, Washington, D. C., 1967, Vols. 1 and 2.

12. Saward, E. W.: The relevance of prepaid group practice to the effective delivery of health services. The New Physician, January 18, 1969.

13. Greenlick, R.: The impact of prepaid group practice on American medical care: A critical evaluation. Annals of the American Academy of Political and Social Science; The Nation's Health: Some Issues 399:100-113, January 1972.

14. Donabedian, A.: An evaluation of prepaid group practice. Inquiry 6:3-27, September 1969; Donabedian, A.: A Review of Some Experiences with Prepaid Group Practice. Bureau of Public Health Economics, Research Series No. 12. University of Michigan, School of Public Health, Ann Arbor, Michigan, 1965.

15. Donabedian, Inquiry, op. cit.

16. Freidson, E.: Patients' Views of Medical Practice. Russell Sage Foundation, New York, 1961.

17. Donabedian, Inquiry, op. cit.

18. Pope, C. R., and Greenlick, M.: Determinants of Medical Care Utilization: Selected Preliminary Tables from Household Interview Survey. Unpublished report presented to Kaiser Foundation Oregon Region Research Policy Committee, San Francisco, California, June 21, 1971.

19. Donabedian, Inquiry, op. cit.

20. MacColl, W.: Group Practice and Prepayment of Medical Care. Public Affairs Press, Washington, D.C., 1966.

21. United States Congress, House, H.R. 11728, 92nd Congress, 1st Session: A Bill to Amend the Public Health Service Act to Provide Assistance and Encouragement for the Establishment and Expansion of Health Maintenance Organizations, and for Other Purposes, 1971.

22. Saward, E. W.: Experience with the Recruitment of Physicians to Prepaid
     Group Practice Medical Care Plans. Unpublished presentation to the
     American Public Health Association, 90th Annual Meeting, Miami,
     Florida, October 17, 1962.
23. Cook, W. H.: Profile of the permanente physician, in Somers, A. R. (Ed.):
     The Kaiser-Permanente Medical Care Program: A Symposium. The
     Commonwealth Fund, New York, 1971, p. 104.
24. Smith, D. B., and Metzner, C. A.: Differential perceptions of health care
     quality in a prepaid group practice. Medical Care 8:264-275, July-
     August 1970.
25. Klarman, H.E.: Economic research in group medicine, in New Horizons in
     Health Care: Proceedings of the First International Congress on Group
     Medicine. Wallingford Press Ltd., Winnipeg, 1970, pp. 178-193.
26. Saward, E. W., Blank, J. D., and Greenlick, M.: Documentation of twenty
     years of operation and growth of a prepaid group practice plan. Medical
     Care 6:231-244, May-June, 1968.
27. Bailey, R. M.: Economics of scale in medical practice, in Klarman, H. (Ed.):
     Empirical Studies in Health Economics. The Johns Hopkins Press, Balti-
     more, pp. 255-273.
28. Stevens, C. M.: Physician supply and national health care goals. Industrial
     Relations, A Journal of Economy and Society 10:119-244, May 1971.
29. United States Department of Health, Education, and Welfare, op. cit.
30. Steinwald, C.: Foundations for Medical Care. Blue Cross Reports, Research
     Series 7, Blue Cross Association, Chicago, August 1971.
31. Saward, E. W.: The relevance of the Kaiser-Permanente experience to the
     health services of the Eastern United States. Bulletin of the New York
     Academy of Medicine 46:707-717, September 1970.
32. United States Congress, House, H.R. 11728, op. cit.
33. Wolkstein, I.: Incentive reimbursement and group practice prepayment, in
     Proceedings of the 19th Annual Group Health Institute. Group Health
     Association of America, Washington, D.C., 1969, pp. 92-100; West,
     H.I.: Group practice prepayment plans in the Medicare program.
     American Journal of Public Health 59:624, April 1969; Newman, H. F.:
     II. The impact of Medicare on group practice prepayment plans.
     American Journal of Public Health 59:629, April 1969.
34. Goldstein, G., Paradise, J., Neil, M., and Wolfe, J.: Experiences in providing
     care to poverty populations, in Proceedings of the 19th Annual Group
     Health Institute, op. cit., p. 74.
35. Colombo, T., Saward, E., and Greenlick, M.: The integration of an OEO
     health program into a prepaid comprehensive group practice plan.
     American Journal of Public Health 59:641, April 1969.
36. Greenlick, M.: Medical service to poverty groups, in Somers, op. cit., p. 138.
37. Colombo, Saward and Greenlick, op. cit., pp. 641-650.
38. Danielson, J. M. (Director, Department of Health Services & Teaching Hos-

pitals, Association of American Medical Colleges): Personal communication, July 14, 1971.

39. Saward, E. W.: Some caveats for medical schools, in Somers, op. cit., pp. 183-188.

40. United States Department of Health, Education, and Welfare: A Study of National Health Insurance Proposals introduced in the 92nd Congress: A Supplementary Report to the Congress. Washington, D.C., July 1971.

41. Williams, E. T.: Speech given at the American Hospital Association Convention, Chicago, August 1971.

Health Care Delivery Systems for Tomorrow: Possibilities and Guidelines*

MADELEINE LEININGER, R.N., PH.D.

HEALTH CARE AS A SOCIETAL IMPERATIVE

Health care is an expected, essential, and important societal imperative in our culture. Accordingly, the American people are becoming increasingly vocal about and dependent upon the need for more, better, and quality-based health services. Americans contend that health services must be made accessible to all who desire or need health care. These societal imperatives are clear and challenging, but they are becoming such pervasive expectations that one wonders if health practitioners can keep pace with the demand. Health educators, practitioners, and administrators are feeling these societal demands and determining ways to cope with these societal expectations, using available manpower and technological and financial resources.

Change is inevitable and essential to meet these societal imperatives. What changes will be needed to provide effective health care delivery services for the immediate future? Are major or minor changes needed to meet societal needs? I believe that some fairly major and substantive changes are necessary to provide effective and accessible health care delivery services for tomorrow. In making major changes, conflicts, challenges, and problems must be expected at the outset. Health educators, practitioners, and administrators should be prepared to deal with conflicts and problems related to substantive kinds of change in order to provide what Americans expect in health care. We need to try and think anew, think openly, and think creatively to change some of our past thought and practice patterns. Changing institutional patterns and modes of health care is a difficult and sizable task as health care is now the second largest industry in this country, and as such it is well institutionalized in our society with many established practices. Instituting any new or

*Originally published in *Health of the Nation* 5, Summer Lecture Series Proceedings, University of Minnesota Hospitals, "The Summer of 1972—Perspectives and Patterns," 1973, pp. 24-31. Reprinted by permission.

novel modes of health care will require creative thinkers, fearless and competent implementors, and objective evaluators. One can suspect that even with the most dynamic, ambitious, and creative designers for, and implementors of new kinds of health care delivery systems for tomorrow, there will probably be only moderate changes as it is quite difficult to change cultural and institutional patterns of health behavior in a drastic way. Normative values and practices of institutionalized health care are generally well-established so that changing these institutionalized patterns requires considerable time, patience, and perseverent goal efforts. I, too, must hasten to add, that before making major changes we need to consider some of the traditional health practices, as some may have positive merits and need to be considered in any newly conceived health care delivery plans. Let us hope, however, that some of the dysfunctional, outdated, and ineffective health practices will be discarded, and be discarded without retaining them for a long period of time. Perpetuating such practices is often costly, time consuming, and energy wasting. Thus, all of us must be prepared to relinquish some of our old dysfunctional or ineffective health practices and beliefs as we adopt new modalities of health care for tomorrow.

MAN'S PAST AND PRESENT HEALTH EMPHASES:
PREVENTATIVE AND RESTORATIVE

In studying man's health behavior from an anthropological perspective, one finds that man's health needs have varied through time and according to social, economic, cultural, political, and environmental factors. However, man's past and present health needs can be classified into two general categories, namely, *restorative needs* and *preventative needs*. Through time, persons assuming various health care roles have developed both informal and formal means to meet man's restorative and preventative health needs.

Interestingly, early man appeared to rely more upon the ways to *prevent* illness than ways to restore health. This is understandable as early man was keenly aware that he needed to protect himself from many unexpected and major life-threatening forces such as monstrous animals, hostile intruders, uncertain weather conditions, changing physical and social environment, and many other kinds of hazards that threatened early man's survival. Ways to prevent sickness, disability, and death must have dominated early man's thinking and mode of living as he moved in and out of precarious and different kinds of environments. Early man was forced to protect and defend himself the best he could, and at all times. Prevention of illness and maintenance of survival was a major life style of early man's thoughts and actions.

Much later in our history, scientifically oriented man was noticeably interested in ways to *restore* his health and there appeared to be less interest in the prevention of illnesses. Scientifically oriented man sought ways to get relief from pain, illness, and emotional anguish, and to have his body parts repaired or replaced. The demands for scientific and effective restorative health care services have been clearly evident with modern man. Moreover, he expects a wide gamut of restorative health services to be readily available to him and to be effective in rapidly curing him of distresses. This theme of restoration to health has dominated the health field until recently.

Most recently, however, one can note the growing tendency that people in our society are seeking ways to *prevent* illness, pain, mental and social anguish. Consequently, prevention is gaining increasing emphasis and is becoming more and more evident through mass communication media and in written publications. Today's prevention theme, however, differs slightly from early man's emphases in that the latter stressed immediate survival, and modern man is primarily interested in avoiding undue pain, prolonged illnesses, and the consequences of chronic deformities or disabilities. More and more, man today wants to limit physical, mental, or social handicaps in order that he can freely live and participate actively in open style of living. He wants to use leisure time to the fullest, and for a long period of time. Illness, pain, and disabilities are often viewed as demoralizing, frustrating, anxiety-producing, and a great social handicap to modern man. In addition, illness and disabilities are very costly, and generally, only the middle and upper classes in our society can economically pay for health services. The American public also knows that health personnel can use "scientifically tested" health measures to prevent illness. Some Americans are willing to spend considerable amounts of money for relief of pain, and to use new medicines and treatments as they become available. The emphases upon prevention is gaining momentum so that in the next two decades health care personnel will be expected to be prevention specialists and generalists. Because of economic losses, social inadequacies, political liabilities (the recent national political situation is an example of this point), changes in religious beliefs, and many psychological concerns all support the need to prevent illness now and in the immediate future. The need is clearly evident to move rapidly in the development of new kinds of preventative health care systems to meet the present societal expectation. This is a challenge, but also a concern, as health professionals have not particularly emphasized prevention in health care services as much as the treatment and the post-illness caring for people.

Of major concern in prevention are the following critical questions:

1. Do we have a systematized body of knowledge on prevention to provide prevention practices?
2. Is there sufficient tested knowledge to develop intervention models to prevent illnesses and illness stresses of a life-threatening nature?
3. In what areas do we feel most secure in offering preventative health services?
4. How valid and reliable are prevention practices in mental health, child care, and cardiac care and other areas, when one considers their application to different cultural and subcultural groups in our society?
5. Will our prevention practices apply to the poor, the affluent, and to people whose life style varies greatly with middle-class Anglo-white people?

These questions and many others need our active consideration. It is my contention that we are on very loose ground in the area of prevention of illness, and especially with different social, economic, and cultural groups. Research efforts and monies are needed to study and verify prevention hunches and practices. New and novel ways to prevent illnesses, using a variety of means, need to be explored. In addition, our nursing, dental, pharmacy, and medical curricula need a major revamping to help students begin to focus upon *prevention* of illnesses, rather than the present pervasive theme of restoring health. This is a major challenge and will require a reorientation in faculty-student thinking. Actually, nurses have been involved for more than a century in health care maintenance and some prevention aspects in helping people in community contexts, and so they can play a major role in helping to identify and test prevention concepts and practices.

SOME SUGGESTED GUIDELINES AND POSSIBILITIES FOR DEVELOPING FUTURE HEALTH CARE DELIVERY SYSTEMS

Unfortunately, limited attention has been given to the philosophy, future goals, and to different models of health care delivery systems for the future. Instead, the focus seems to be upon financing health care without knowing *what* we will be financing and the *rationale* for the projected money expenditures. Our first task should be to explore and study different conceptual models of health care delivery for the future with consideration of the financial, human resources and service consequences for each model. For example, the "open-client-centered" health care delivery model developed by the author is based upon an open maintenance system health care with restorative and *preventative* subsystems of care and with focus upon ways to accommodate community needs.[1] This is one model to consider, but we need to think of other types of models and theories of future health care delivery in our society.

In addition, we need to face squarely and openly some realistic problems of our present health care delivery systems if we expect to use facets of them. We must look at their purposes, organizational structure, management, and use and abuse of human and technological resources. Thus, in this section, I will highlight some of the major barriers and possibilities which I feel we need to examine as we develop and plan for new or modified health care delivery models for the future. Fortunately, during the past 25 years as a nurse-practitioner, educator, social scientist, and humanist, I have been able to experience and study some of these critical problems and the possibilities for different kinds of health care services. My comments will be candid and critical in order to help us begin to think anew about areas we may fear or are reluctant to examine.

First, in the future we must develop *open types* of health care delivery systems in which Americans can get health care services quickly, effectively, and with less red tape. Currently, one of the most serious major problems with our present health care delivery modes is that people get discouraged and lost in obtaining health care. This is due to many factors but primarily, I contend, due to the fact that we have actually a *closed type* of health care systems. Our health care systems are closed because they are largely controlled, regulated, and financially monitored by one professional group, namely the medical profession.[2] In keeping with the principles and theory of general systems, one will find that closed systems prove to be dead systems in time. Closed systems presently function in a fairly isolated, controlled, and insulated concept without full use of available resources—human and material. With our present closed health systems, consumers are expected to enter and leave the health system (whatever form it may be) under a fairly tight controlled system and under the ultimate control of the medical profession. Interestingly, but true, in our American culture, children and adults are expected to enter and leave the health care system under the control of a physician. The medical profession does dominate and control our health practices. As Freidson states[3]

> . . . professions in general and medicine in particular cannot live up to their professed ideas as long as they possess thorough growing autonomy to control the terms and content of their work and as long as they are dominant in the division of labor. In essence, I suggested ways by which professional dominance and autonomy could be tempered by administrative accountability, by accountability to the individual patient himself, and by the deliberate encouragement of workers who can compete with the medical practitioner.

From an anthropological perspective, there are few cultures in the world in which people are so tightly regulated and socially sanctioned by one discipline. Moreover, our financial plans (past and still today) continue to support a closed system of operation in that all health payments sooner or later seem to be funneled through and need the signature or payment of a physician (or their designated). For years, nurses have provided direct health services to clients, and yet it is still virtually impossible for this large and predominantly female group to get direct payments, except for a small amount through private duty nursing. Primary, secondary, or tertiary payments such as direct payments from Medicare, Medicaid, Blue Cross, Blue Shield and private insurance plans are still largely funneled through physicians' hands for clients to receive care services. Most of our national health insurance companies continue to perpetuate this closed financial system which leads to a closed type of health care service. This approach limits the consumer's use of other health providers' services whose services are different and usually substantive in nature. Most importantly, other health professional groups could reach people at an early point with their health care stresses or concerns and provide preventative and restorative services—thus preventing illnesses from being serious and more costly to remedy at a later time.

I firmly believe that the future health care systems in our society must be developed as open systems in which clients do have the freedom and opportunity to choose and pay their health practitioner of choice, and according to the kind of service they want and can recieve. I believe such an open health care system would revolutionize our health care delivery services and could provide greater access to a variety of health practitioners who could help people when they need help, and thus avoid unnecessary delays in getting health care. Currently, there are qualified health professionals who could serve in a front line position to prevent illness and to provide health counseling to people who need such help. This approach could greatly reduce serious illnesses and avoid costly hospitalization for a number of people.

Moreover, with an open health system approach, there would be greater emphasis in responding to new inputs from within and outside the health care system. It would require that we become more sensitive to clients' needs, the community needs, and the community resources. An open health system would fully use *all* health professional resources and distribute responsibilities and areas of accountability according to client and community needs. In addition, there would be greater participation of community people in health maintenance and control of health programs.

Second, our health care delivery systems of tomorrow must have *more knowledge and research inputs from the social sciences and the humanities than presently exist.* As a nurse-social scientist, I find our present health organizations and health systems need to be urgently reassessed and reevaluated in light of our present research findings and knowledge from the social sciences. To date, we have limitedly drawn upon social science research findings and approaches in developing and maintaining health organizational structures and systems. This is perhaps one major reason why our health systems have failed or become ineffective. Historically, our health organizations and practices have been predominantly conceptualized as biological science models or organismic models. Most of them have evolved as a "cell growth model" with limited awareness of social and humanistic factors. Since health organizational structures are exceedingly complex, it is difficult for many of them to survive on such organismic models. By and large our health organizations across the country have "grown like Topsy" and without the benefit of social science research and substantive knowledge inputs from social scientists and humanists. Accordingly, one finds that our health organizations are showing symptoms of psychosocial pathology which are reflected in these commonly heard public statements: "depersonalization of care," "fragmentation of our human needs," "poor utilization of available health personnel," "no health system or structure at all," "a tightly controlled and rigid system of care," "limited consideration of the client as a person and more of an object," "inefficient use of interdisciplinary staff," and "poor organization to get health services quickly and efficiently." These statements and others reflect the urgent need for social science and humanistic inputs into future health care delivery systems. It is, indeed, a pity that the social science research theories and principles have hardly been tapped for they might have saved us from today's health care dilemma.

I believe that the predominant exclusion of social science content is largely due to our traditional emphases in the health fields upon the biological nature of man and with only token kind of lip-service regarding man's social and psychocultural needs. If we pause to examine medical school catalogs across the country, we find that more than two-thirds of the curricula are focused upon the biological science courses. Although many nursing curricula tend to follow medical school curricula (and especially in the early days), there has generally been more emphases in nursing from its early beginnings to focus upon man's psychosocial needs. Then, with the advent of collegiate nursing education, there has been greater effort to balance content from the natural sciences, social sciences, and the humanities in order to obtain a holistic view of man's health needs. But currently, much of the available cultural and social knowledges and research is not fully recognized or used in the health sciences. Our consumers, however, are expecting health personnel to give more attention to their cultural, social, political, legal, economic, and humanistic needs. Consequently, social forces are providing the impetus for changes.

Interestingly, many physicians directing our health centers today have had scanty to virtually no preparation in dealing with complex organizational systems and social system behavior, and yet they are expected to provide effective leadership to people in these kinds of social systems. Frequently, a biological specialist, endocrinologist, surgeon, or similar specialist is responsible for these large and complex health institutions. Granted that physicians have considerable political and financial power, this may not be sufficient to cope with organizational problems or to be knowledgeable organizational change agents to modify health systems. Today there are a growing number of nurse-scientists and some social workers who have advanced preparation in organizational theory and practices, but since they are women they often are not considered for these top administrative positions to date. In contrast, male nurse-social scientists are being sought after and employed in these leadership positions. Thus sex discrimination practices in the top health administration positions still need to be recognized and remedied.

Third, our future health care systems must offer *a variety of health care services and systems to meet our pluralistic societal needs.* Presently, our health services are limited in meeting diverse cultural, economic, and social group needs. Moreover, our health delivery systems are largely *hospital-centered,* and perceived as *the* key means of meeting societal health needs, rather than recognizing that the hospital is *one* of many possible means to meet the diverse needs of people in our society. Most of our health care delivery institutions have been located in metropolitan urban areas and only a few health facilities are located in rural areas, which limits care to many sectors of our diverse population groups. Future health care delivery systems must provide a *variety* of health care services to *meet* a variety of our people's needs and in different key geographical locations.

Some new and promising varieties of health care services which need to be considered in the future include: (1) "mini" short-term ambulatory care services; (2) "maxi" long-term ambulatory care services; (3) crisis and on-going health instruction services; (4) crisis counseling services; (5) primary, first-line care services; (6) preventative care services; (7) self-care services; (8) family care clinics; (9) mental health "worried-person" services; (10) sociocultural health services; and others.

Many of the evolving and current ambulatory and primary care programs which are mushrooming across the country are very exciting and offer encouraging possibilities, as well as the new kinds of emergency short-term care services. These services and their concomitant systems should continue to be developed with explicit criteria in mind such as the means to: (1) increase the *accessibility* of health services to people at an early time; (2) provide *continuity* of health services; (3) *prevent* serious illnesses, disabilities, deformities or complications; (4) provide *community-based* health services; (5) reduce *service costs* because of early interventions; (6) maximize use of *available health manpower* resources, especially nursing services.

Most importantly, future health care systems must develop ways to *meet and/or accommodate the needs of different cultural, social, and economic groups.* We need to give more thought, however, to the health needs of people with different cultural backgrounds such as the Chicano peoples, the Afro-Americans, the Blacks, the American Indian groups, the Orientals, and to many other cultural and subcultural groups in our society. Subcultural groups such as the poor, affluent, drug and alcohol users, rural, urban, suburban, religious cults, and other groups must be considered in health service planning programs. All these groups have identifiable health needs, norms, beliefs, and practices, which often do not receive sufficient attention.[4] Again, research findings and knowledge from the social sciences could help us build sound types of health care programs for these cultural groups, ranging from the least acculturated, to those more fully acculturated.

Responding to, and planning with people of different group and cultural orientations, necessitates that we recognize the cultural values and practices between the *native health value systems* and our *professional health value system.* From my own research, I have found that these two health systems are conceptually and operationally quite different and sometimes need to be treated as two different value systems. When health personnel fail to recognize that indigenous health groups do have their own health systems, it is difficult to be helpful to cultural groups. Conflicts and problems arise and can limit effectiveness in helping others. As we recognize cultural norm differences (as well as some of the similarities), then we can make linkages between different cultural groups and those of professional cultural systems. In my view, I believe it may take the decade of the 1970s to accomplish this goal and to develop theories and health care practices that facilitate interprofessional and native health care working relationships and structures. It is, however, an exciting and critical challenge which I believe will provide some new ideas about health care delivery systems not yet known. I believe it will help us see other ways to deliver health care to people and to change aspects of our current health systems operations. The comparative frame of reference is invaluable to health personnel to see new dimensions of health behavior. An attitude of learning from others and placing some credibility to what people do and say over time, and in crises situations, is essential to this approach. Hence, a variety of health care delivery systems and subsystems needs to be developed to serve people in our pluralistic society.

Fourth, health care delivery systems of the future must become *more community- and client-centered* than presently found. Today, many of our health services tend to be focused upon the norms and practices of a designated health institution, a particular hospital, or a particular professional group. All too frequently, the individual client, family, or social group needs receive less attention with normative practices of institutions overriding the individual or community concerns. The client's social or cultural background and his particular community setting, with its own life style for health maintenance, need more attention. The actual and potential health resources of a given community may be barely recognized or known to some health professional practitioners. Thus, in planning future health care delivery modes, we must obtain *grass-roots* information about the community or communities which health professionals will serve and to show a genuine interest in the client's community.

Another important consideration is to recognize the needs of *clients-from-a-distance,* that is, people who come to health institutions from distant communities. With modern modes of transportation and communication, we can anticipate that clients will come from distant communities and countries of which we have very little knowledge, such as those clients from Africa, the Pacific Islands, and many other "non-Western" settings. How can we develop health care systems to accommodate the needs of people from significantly different kinds of Western and non-Western health-oriented communities? How can we help health personnel respond in a helpful and effective way to people who come from *entirely* different communities and who often have markedly different health styles, health norms, and practices? Do we superimpose our health values upon them? Unfortunately, only a small core of social scientists and health practitioners are looking at these very important, timely, and critical questions for tomorrow's health care delivery systems. With our rapidly changing and developing world community focus, travel modes, current technology and mass communication media, it is urgent to consider these aspects in developing transcultural health systems. In sum, both client- and community-centered health systems and transcultural health systems programs need to be developed now to provide realistic, humanistic, and personalized community health services to people.

Fifth, I believe that future health care delivery systems must give serious thought to the *concepts and practices related to role complementarity and new role reorientations.* By role complementarity, I am referring to the cognitive linkage or blending together of the skills and knowledges of *different* health disciplines in order to help clients benefit in a maximal way from each discipline's contribution. Currently, there is a growing trend to assume and/or plan that all health disciplines now and in the future become alike. The line of thinking seems to go in this manner: All health needs of people are basically the same. All health disciplines should have a similar focus. Therefore, all health disciplines should be prepared alike and be ready to respond to similar health needs of people. Accordingly, the dominant themes of *role uniformity, role conformity,* and *role likeness* are being promoted in some health centers. While I would firmly support the idea that there are core or common health area needs which all disciplines need to understand, it is my position that *each* health discipline does have some fairly special, unique, and different kinds of contributions and domains of foci to offer health consumers.[5] It would, therefore, be most unfortunate to lump or dump everyone into a uni-health discipline and be content to have the same focus. To support the beginning signs of a "uni-health science discipline" I believe would be unfortunate, inefficient, unwise, and it would seriously limit providing clients with the different kinds of health services and care needs. Actually, health consumers do expect different areas as they receive health services from different health disciplines. It is important to recognize these differences and to maintain professional pride in the contributions of each discipline to health care services. For example, it would be unfortunate to see the discipline of medicine relinquish its traditional and important emphases upon physical pathology, disease conditions, and illness behavior. As a health consumer, I would expect physicians to be highly knowledgeable and skilled in these domains of expertise. I, too, would expect physical and occupational therapists to remain primarily knowledgeable and skilled in their respective areas of emphases and expertise. Accordingly, I expect the discipline of nursing to emphasize its central and dominant emphases upon direct and on-going health care services to people which stresses support, nurturance, comfort, rehabilitation, health counseling, and education measures. Role complementarity, rather than role likeness, is needed for tomorrow's health systems. *The blending together of different health disciplines, expertise, and interests is the critical challenge of the future.* I believe that interdiscipline role complementarity is taking shape, but it needs much more openness in communication, feelings, viewpoints, and open planning together. We, too, need what I call "interdiscipline confrontations" in which the different health disciplines openly and frankly discuss their viewpoints, feelings, hang-ups, and concerns with one another to provide empathetic and realistic working relationships. Victorian politeness and undue deference toward superiors as well as subjugated cooperation practices need to be replaced with open and honest confrontation sessions among health disciplines in our efforts to achieve true interdisciplinary and complementary role relationships.

The present federal and national push to prepare many health care workers under the label of "physician assistants" who will be assuming very similar role activities to that of the professional nurse is, in my view, a waste of the taxpayers' money. It appears to be a duplication of professional efforts and largely a sexual discrimination problem. Currently, a mass of physician assistants of a variety of kinds are being prepared in short-term, 3 to 6-month programs instead of utilizing a core of well-qualified nurses who are prepared to do comparable role activities. But since the nursing profession is largely female, the professional nurse is being cast aside and instead, a core of men is being prepared. As already evident by a number of perceptive physicians, nurses, and consumers, many of these short-term assistants do not measure up to professional nurses' knowledge and skills which have been acquired in substantive 3 to 5-year programs. The professional nurse has great capabilities *if* the sex barrier and interdisciplinary problems can be alleviated.

Role reorientation must also be considered as role behaviors and expectations between disciplines evolve. In any open and dynamic health system that is responsive to societal needs, role functions and activities do change and so do interrole relationships. Different health disciplines must be prepared to extend, change, and modify role relationships and expectations to meet societal needs. Our role activities or tasks need be dropped to accommodate new or expanded activities and functions. To achieve role reorientation one needs time to identify, discuss, and become fully aware of the nature and consequences of role changes. Thus, role complementarity and role reorientation are critical considerations for future health care delivery practices. Role uniformity and role conformity will not support a viable health care delivery system in the future. We need open, dynamic, and changing structural flexibility in our systems.

Sixth, future health care systems must give more emphasis to *prevention* and to *primary care health services.* Since this aspect was discussed earlier in this paper, it will not be explored further. It is my view, however, that the nurses' contribution to primary care and to prevention can and should be substantive in nature because of their professional preparation and long-term experiences in the community. Many of our collegiate-prepared nurses are prepared to understand and respond to clients in a variety of community settings. Their scientific and humanistic backgrounds are invaluable to move them into primary health care programs. Some nurses have been fairly quick and adept to observe and assess the preventative and primary needs of people. As the nurse develops more confidence she can do what she has been largely prepared to do; then she will be more effective in primary care. In many settings nurses are engaged in outreach primary care programs with families, groups, and individuals and are taking more responsibility for health care assessments, planning, and follow-up care.[6,7,8]

The nurse is capable of building and expanding upon her general nursing skills. Individual and group support from nursing educators and service administration is needed to encourage nurses to move into primary nurse care practices. The professional nurse generalist is no foreign person to people in many communities and this is an important advantage to many physician assistants who have limited previous professional community-based experiences and often limited preparation in community services in their programs. Both social workers and community-based nurses are presently crucial resources for the development of our future health care delivery systems. Of course, the nurse practitioner will continue to help clients with acute and chronic care problems as she helps people with their preventative and restorative health needs. It is time we fully utilize the nurse's skills and potentialities and we will then be able to reduce the number of many new kinds of short-term prepared assistant practitioners. I believe the latter will be short-lived as they do not have sufficient background to cope with the wide variety and highly complex kinds of health care problems which clients expect of professional health practitioners of today and tomorrow. I , too, believe there is a real danger of having an oversupply of these paraprofessional or allied health workers who require fairly close supervision and guidance. Currently, some professional nurses are supervising and teaching these workers which may be limiting the nurse's time and energy in giving direct and primary nursing care to people.

In future health care delivery modes, we must provide opportunities for both collaborative and for independent interdisciplinary role activities. This is essential to support each discipline's expertise, to promote professional growth, and to nurture efficient and effective use of health personnel. Models of interdiscipline collaboration and fairly independent professional practices need to be studied and explored in new health care delivery systems for effective and efficient use of health disciplines.

Seventh, in developing future health care delivery modalities, *more thought and more enticements (or rewards) must be given to health disciplines who live and work in rural communities, small towns, and in isolated outreach areas.* Small groups of interdiscipline health workers need to be sent to these areas rather than solo practitioners who soon become overwhelmed with work expectations. Sending one person is an unwise plan as health practitioners need *others* to support and confer with them in their endeavors to meet complex health problems, to reduce feelings of being professionally isolated and alienated, as well as inundated with client's health needs. Rewards must be developed to entice health professionals to remain in these isolated and rural communities.

Finally, it is well known that *cost* factors must be considered as a guideline to the future development of health care delivery systems, but since costs of health have been the major public focus, I will not add further comments here. Instead, I shall mention that means for *quality control* must be an important guideline. This can only be achieved by effective evaluation schemes for all emerging and new health care delivery systems. Evaluation means must be built in at the beginning to help us answer the question: What difference does it make if we do 'x,' 'y' or 'z'?

In this presentation, I have identified and briefly discussed some of the key considerations and possibilities for developing, designing, and implementing new health care delivery modes for the immediate future. To be sure, there are other areas; however, these are some of the relevant and important considerations for the future. The path to changes is never a smooth, definitive, or clear one. Frankness, honesty, and openness in what needs to be changed are essential. Open communication in our discussions among health disciplines and with consumers cannot be overemphasized. Courage, creativeness, and determination to change that which needs to be changed for a better health care delivery system for tomorrow are essential for the important and sizable task ahead.

REFERENCES

1. Leininger, Madeleine: An open health care system mode. Nursing Outlook 21:171-175, March 1973.
2. Ibid.
3. Freidson, Eliot: Professional Dominance: The Social Structure of Medical Care. Atherton Press, Inc., New York, 1970.
4. Leininger, Madeleine: Nursing and Anthropology: Two Worlds to Blend. John Wiley and Company, New York, 1971.
5. Leininger, Madeleine: This I believe about interdisciplinary health education for the future. Nursing Outlook 19: 787-791, 1971.
6. Leininger, Madeleine, Little, D. E., and Carnevali, Doris: Primex. American Journal of Nursing 72:1274-1277, July 1972.
7. Norris, Catherine: Direct access to the patient. American Journal of Nursing 70: 1006-1010, May 1970.
8. Lewis, C. E., and Resnik, Barbara A.: Nurse clinics and progressive ambulatory patient care. New England Journal of Medicine 277: 1236-1241, December 1967.

Nurse Practitioners in Primary Care: The McMaster University Educational Program*†

WALTER O. SPITZER, M.D., M.P.H., AND
DOROTHY J. KERGIN, R.N., PH.D.

Summary: In 1971 McMaster University offered an educational program for nurse practitioners sponsored jointly by the Faculty of Medicine and the School of Nursing. Priority in the pilot program was given to nurses employed in family practice settings and to those participating in related McMaster studies. Because of the implications of a change in role for both nurse and physician, one requirement for acceptance of a nurse in the program was participation of the physician-associate in the educational program.

The program prepares registered nurses to extend their responsibilities in primary health care activities for the assessment and management of patients in family practice. The current evaluations of the pilot-study results suggest that such programs can contribute effective resources towards meeting expectations of ready access to primary care by the people of Canada.

RATIONALE

Background. In discussions about health professionals allied to the physician, the realm of ambulatory care[1,2] has been identified for priority in consideration and development. This decision does not deny the fact that for at least two decades health professionals associated with the physician have been effectively and desirably expanding their roles in the hospital setting and in the care of reposing

*Originally published as "Nurse practitioners in primary care, I. The McMaster University educational program," in Canadian Medical Association Journal 108:991-995, April 21, 1973. Reprinted by permission.

†Pilot program supported by the Ontario Health Resources Development Plan of the Ontario Ministry of Health (Project D.M.36).

95

patients. Nor does it overlook the fact that the role of the physician has also changed. The constant, gradual evolutionary process throughout the whole health field can be expected to continue. However, because of the current emphasis and the apparent requirements of the Canadian health-care delivery system in the early seventies, our focus is the delivery of ambulatory health care and particularly primary or first-contact care.

No serious challenge in Canada has arisen to the multidisciplinary consensus[3] that the nurse is the professional most appropriate to assume a broader and better delineated role in ambulatory service and to supplement physician care. Moreover, the deployment of outpost nurses as the principal providers of care has been documented for decades by the Department of National Health and Welfare in remote northern jurisdictions across the country, by the International Grenfell Association in Newfoundland, by the United Church of Canada in British Columbia, and by most provincial health departments.

There has been evidence of a surplus of nurses in Ontario during recent years.[4] The surplus has continued and has been verified through formal study.[5] Ratios of population to physicians in Ontario are now seldom unfavourable except for primary care physicians in non-urban areas.[6] These facts influenced program planners at McMaster University to adopt the following course of action for a nurse-practitioner educational program: only nurses would be enrolled; priority would be given to the development of nurse practitioners in primary care (family practice nurses); and in the long run, preference for admission to the educational program would be given to candidates residing in underserviced areas and committed to return to those areas.

The appropriate Councils and Committees of the Division of Health Sciences at McMaster University concurred with the consensus among nurses, physicians and others that there was no need in Canada to develop a new category of worker called "physician assistant."[7]

Consequently, a new Canadian Educational Program for Nurse Practitioners was established during 1971. The program was operated with joint sponsorship of the Faculty of Medicine and the School of Nursing and funded by the Ontario Ministry of Health. On February 2, 1972, the first 22 graduates were awarded Certificates by the Division of Health Sciences and the School of Adult Education to signify their attainment of the educational objectives of the program.*

This paper presents an account of the conceptual framework of a university educational program for nurse practitioners. We shall also describe the instructional objectives of the curriculum, the method of implementation and the strategy of evaluation.

---

*At the time that McMaster's first class of nurse practitioners qualified in December 1971, one other comparable program (Community Nurse Program) had begun (September 1971) at the University of Montreal. Six other universities in four provinces had definite plans to sponsor projects with target dates for launching in early 1972. The goal of all proposed programs was to prepare nurses for northern outpost assignments; the combined annual enrolment for the seven projects other than that described in this paper was to be 38. Dalhousie University initiated its two-year course leading to credentials in midwifery and outpost nursing in 1967; this is well known as Canada's first program for outpost nurses.

Conceptual Framework. The gradual process of change in the health field is occasionally punctuated by deliberate, explicit definition of roles of health professionals. In redefining the role of the nurse in ambulatory care, we recognized the importance of one particular criterion in classifying workers allied to the physician*—the exercise of clinical judgement. By this criterion we distinguish true health professionals from technicians. Examples of the former are psychologists, social workers and physiotherapists. Examples of the latter are operating-room technicians, ophthalmic assistants and inhalation therapists. The technical personnel are generally oriented to implement decisions resulting from the clinical judgement exercised by another health professional.

We believe that the exercise of clinical judgement is the characteristic that best discriminates the nurse practitioner from the individual who serves as a technician or managerial assistant to the physician. To acquire clinical judgement a nurse must enhance her ability to assess the need for care and to plan care. This is accomplished by augmenting her skills in data gathering and problem solving. We view the proposed designation "physician assistant" for any worker who meets the criterion of a true health professional as inappropriate and perhaps misleading.

Depending on the setting where they work, nurses with redefined roles in primary care develop distinctive emphasis in their patterns of practice. They may work in close association with physicians in family practices where patients are usually exposed to both the nurse and the physician in individual episodes of care. Most nurse practitioners (or family practice nurses) who have graduated from the McMaster Program now practice in this way. On the other hand, a nurse may be the principal purveyor of primary care services in underserviced areas. In that capacity the nurse works with considerable professional independence in discharging most of her responsibilities. The Report of the Committee on Nurse Practitioners[8] used the term "physician surrogate" to describe this category because many of her activities (sometimes including midwifery) are ordinarily performed only by physicians in other geographic areas. Such nurses are usually designated "outpost nurses."

As will become apparent in the description of skills and knowledge required of nurse practitioner graduates, we do not advocate that they become "junior physicians." The nurse's abilities are augmented to encompass an appropriately delineated scope of responsibility and authority for the clinical management of patients. The McMaster nurse practitioner learns to assess patients in a manner that leads to a correct action decision, regardless of whether or not it always leads to a precise diagnosis. Three broad categories of action decisions are: (a) recommendation of a specific treatment, (b) no intervention other than reassurance, and (c) referral to the associated physician.

The definition of the nurse practitioner developed for the program is as follows:

A nurse practitioner (family practice nurse) is a nurse in an expanded role

---

*Excluded from this scheme of classification are support staff who do not have differentiated skills oriented to health care (e.g. janitors, clerks, typists, etc.).

oriented to the provision of primary health care as a member of a team of health professionals, relating to families on a long-term basis and who, through a combination of special education and experience beyond a baccalaureate degree or a diploma, is qualified to fulfil the expectations of this role.[9,10]

Key Principles Influencing Adopted Educational Policy.

1. The orientation of the curriculum should emphasize the nurse's development of added skills in clinical problem solving. An orientation that is primarily procedural is undesirable.

2. To develop nurse practitioners by an apprentice system would handicap assessment of the nurse's performance and might impair the evolution of desirable patterns of practice. Therefore the education of nurse practitioners should take place in post-secondary institutions. Reasonable comparability between educational programs should be sought within provincial or national jurisdictions.

3. The educational program should be interdisciplinary. Faculties of medicine and nursing should be jointly deployed; nurses should learn new skills together with physicians who learn new roles.

IMPLEMENTATION

Planning and Execution. Planning for the Nurse Practitioner Educational Program began in July 1970, when a Sub-Committee on Primary Care Education was formed to develop a continuing education program for nurses employed in family physicians' offices.[11] The Committee, consisting of nurses, physicians (educators and practitioners) and a social worker, together with a full-time nurse educator, was responsible for guiding the program through the developmental and operational phases. Four student representatives joined the Committee when the program began.

Admission Procedures and Criteria. In January 1971 it was agreed that applications for the Nurse Practitioner Program would be received from nurses associated with practices participating in several collaborative research studies involving nurses and physicians in family practice settings. Criteria for admission of a nurse to the program were defined as follows:

1. Current registration with the College of Nurses of Ontario.
2. Employment in the office of a family physician or in a family health-care centre.
3. Participation of the associated physician in the program.

All applicants (physicians and nurses) were interviewed by the Admissions Committee to ensure mutual commitment to the concepts of the teaching program. Required of the physician was agreement to participate in "on-campus" sessions and to serve as a preceptor when the nurse was practising her newly learned skills. When screening had been completed 27 nurses were accepted. Four nurses withdrew in March when the Family Medicine Unit in which they were to have been employed failed to develop financial support. One other nurse withdrew from the course in June. The remaining 22 nurses completed the program successfully.

Curriculum. The curriculum was designed to assist the nurses to develop the following categories of skills and knowledge:

1. Interviewing and history-taking.
2. Physical examination.
3. Pre- and postnatal care.
4. Well-child assessment and advisement.
5. Evaluation and management of common acute and chronic disorders.
6. Evaluation and management of common emotional disorders.
7. Evaluation and management of common disorders of the family unit.
8. Geriatrics—assessment and advisement.
9. Utilization of community health and welfare services.

Since the students were being prepared to function as first-contact health professionals, heavy emphasis was given to distinguishing the normal from the abnormal. The fact that the distinction between normality and abnormality is often equivocal and arbitrary was stressed, as was the need for continued assessment of criteria of normality and abnormality. The student was not expected to diagnose different kinds of "abnormality."

Teaching and Learning Methods. The course involved some full-time and mainly part-time activities for a calendar year. The program could be conducted, if given full-time, in four months of classroom instruction and an additional three to four months of clinical work.*

The program began in February 1971 and continued through to December. It was a work-study program—the nurses continued to work in their home practices, attending classes or tutorials for four to eight hours each Wednesday except during March, when they were full-time students at the university. During the winter and spring segments of the program the basic methods of learning were: (a) instruction in small groups, (b) seminars, (c) lecture/discussions, (d) clinical practice, and (e) individualized self-learning, utilizing library and audiovisual resources. The students met each Wednesday afternoon to discuss problems and topics of general interest to all the group. Small group tutorials dealt with application of knowledge and skills, the problems of attitudes and roles, barriers to achievement of objectives, and integration of subject matter.

The fall session followed a summer of sharpening of skills and clarifying of roles in the "home" practices. In the fall each student was an active participant in the preparation and presentation of two sessions. This experience enabled students to learn more about specific content areas and to become familiar with different kinds and uses of resource materials for solving patients' problems.

---

*The continuing permanent program is now being given as four months' full-time instruction on campus plus four months' supervised practice experience.

Once monthly, the family physicians with whom the nurses worked attended the Wednesday sessions. These sessions were especially designed to facilitate the role change process and to assist the nurses and physicians engaged in rendering primary health care to better understand their complementary responsibilities and abilities.

At the time of the mid-term evaluations in June, it was found that most students had great difficulty in carrying out a physical assessment and in organizing the information gathered. To overcome these problems, hospital rounds were scheduled one-half day per week for 12 weeks during the fall term, six weeks with a pediatrician and six weeks with an internist. These in-hospital experiences also served to focus the nurses' attention on events that had brought patients for admission to hospital and to permit discussion of the primary care nurse's and physician's roles in continuing management of the observed patients.

Each student also spent a half-day session in a home for the elderly. This additional experience was designed to assist the nurses to develop a perspective on ageing and chronic illness useful in planning care, to form a clearer conception of the complex picture of chronic illness, and to deal with patients' problems one by one.

Evaluation of Students. Various techniques were used to evaluate the students. Common to all was the goal of determining whether the candidates successfully attained the pre-established standards of professional behaviour as set forth by the instructional objectives.

Because this was a pilot program, at least one third of the examiners and evaluators (nurses and physicians) were external. They were either private practitioners, not based in McMaster-affiliated hospitals, or colleagues from other Canadian health-science university faculties and from professional associations.

Evaluation techniques included (a) a written examination, including multiple-choice, short answer and clinical problem-solving questions; (b) ongoing evaluation by tutor-supervisors; and (c) oral and practical evaluations.

The greatest emphasis was placed on the last two forms of assessment. In particular, the oral practical evaluations seemed to discriminate well between levels of competency among students. Three such evaluations were conducted during the course. Although certain modifications were made each time, the basic format was as follows:

1. Each student conducted an interview and physical assessment of a real patient, in the presence of two examiners, a nurse and a physician.

2. Immediately afterwards, each student and the examining team viewed a 10-minute videotaped case presentation of a simulated (or instructed) patient.

3. The student then discussed the real and simulated patients with the examiners, describing her evaluation of the presenting problem and recommendations for action.

4. The student's performance was scored according to standardized marking sheets.

5. After each individual student evaluation, a McMaster faculty member met with evaluators and then with the student to interpret the examiners' report.

This mechanism was used to provide consistency throughout the evaluations, as well as to provide immediate constructive "feedback" for the students and faculty. To facilitate recall of the evaluation, all evaluative sessions were audio-tape recorded. The tapes and copies of the examiners' reports were later made available to the students for individual review.

Of the 23 students who enrolled initially, 22 attempted the first-term assessments and 20 were successful. In the final evaluations 22 students fulfilled the overall criteria. Two students were deficient in two sections of the curriculum as determined in "paper and pencil tests." However, they were granted a satisfactory overall rating because they had demonstrated their abilities effectively in an "action setting" corresponding to the same categories in the first-term evaluations.

Costs. Total cost of the program excluding evaluation was $69,420, an average of $3100 per successful graduate. The amount granted by the Ontario Health Resources Development Plan (OHRDP) of the Ministry of Health was $40,192 or 60%. The balance represents faculty contributions of McMaster University. The cost of evaluating the program ($17,700) included 90% support from OHRDP.

CONTINUING EVALUATION

On-going semi-formal surveillance of the graduates is under way. Records are being kept to document whether the nurse practitioners are practising or not, in what modality, in what setting and in what geographic location. Informal contacts and continuing educational activities for alumni will facilitate data gathering.

Four formal studies will provide more rigorous evidence for the effects of the nurse-practitioner concept upon family physicians, nurses and patients.

In the first of the series the instrument and methodology for assessing the activities and role expectations of the nurse were developed. The project, entitled "A Study of the Nurse Activities in Primary Care Settings,"[12] is a description of the activities of nurses employed in a sample of 50 family physicians' offices within the Hamilton region. The conclusions of the study were that nurse activities related to direct patient care involved less than one third of conventional office nurses' time, and almost equal time was devoted to activities that could be carried out by a non-trained nurse alternate or receptionist.

The second project, "The Smithville-McMaster Family Medical Centre Study," has a "before and after" design and, in a semi-rural population of the Niagara peninsula, assesses the impact of a primary care team that incorporates the nurse practitioner. The most important variable assessed is population acceptance of the nurse in the new role.

Two complementary randomized controlled trials of the nurse practitioner have now been concluded. The first trial examines the consequences of the new concept for physicians and nurses. In 14 practices, with physicians' support and commitment to participation, the nurses had applied for enrolment in the educational program. Seven applicants were randomly assigned to an experimental group and admitted to the program, the remaining nurses and practices being retained as controls. This is designated as "The Southern Ontario Randomized Trial of the Nurse Practitioner." The second trial was planned to focus upon the effects on patients. The families of two suburban family-medicine practices were randomly assigned to receive care from nurse practitioners on the one hand or family physicians on the other. This study is known as "The Burlington Randomized Trial of the Nurse Practitioner." The variables under assessment in both foregoing trials include the following: in the patients—functional capacity, medical services' utilization, acceptance of the nurse, and general satisfaction; in the nurses and physicians—alterations in clinical/non-clinical activities and professional attitudes; in quality of care—managerial strategy for "indicator conditions," use of medications and appraisal of referral decisions; and in the practices—growth and profitability. Analysis of the results is nearing completion and results will be reported shortly.

THE FUTURE

The University has given its approval to continuing the program under the joint auspices of the School of Nursing, the Faculty of Medicine and the School of Adult Education. Support for three years has been approved by the Department of National Health and Welfare. This will permit education of at least 100 more nurse practitioners during that time. Priority of admission to the certificate program will be accorded to residents of medically underserviced areas who are committed to serve in such localities. The incorporation of clinical assessment and systematic history-taking skills in the undergraduate B.Sc.N. curriculum and a family practice elective in the final year are now being implemented, as recommended by the Committee on Nurse Practitioners.[13]

Although a firm verdict concerning the effect of nurse practitioners in primary care awaits further evidence from health care trials and other studies, preliminary indicators of satisfaction, acceptance and financial viability suggest that these programs will effectively serve important health care expectations of the population.

ACKNOWLEDGEMENTS

We should like to acknowledge the indispensable role played by Mrs. Joan Davis, the full-time faculty member responsible for the day-to-day administration of the pilot program. We are also indebted to Mr. Mark Magenheim who served as administrative assistant. The program became a reality as a result of extensive contributions of scores of faculty members and community practitioners. Of these, Drs. J. C. Sibley, R. G. McAuley and W. A. M. Russell, Miss Norma A. Wylie and Prof. L. E. Levine invested a very high number of hours in the development of policy and curriculum planning.

REFERENCES

1. Department of National Health and Welfare: National Conference on Assistance to the Physician. Ottawa, April 6-8, 1971.

2. Proceedings of the Workshop on the Role of Allied Professionals in the Delivery of Primary Health Care. Toronto, College of Family Physicians of Canada, 1971.

3. Department of National Health and Welfare: Report of the Committee on Nurse Practitioners (Chairman: Thomas J Boudreau). Ottawa, April 1972, p. 41.

4. Smiley, Jr.: Mobility, Service and Attitudes of Active and Inactive Nurses. A Preliminary Report. Research and Planning Branch, Department of Health, Province of Ontario, December 1968, p. 13.

5. Imai, H. R.: Report of a Preliminary Survey to Explore the Nursing Employment Situation in Canada in Terms of the Number of 1971 Graduates of Canadian Schools of Nursing Registered/Licensed for the First Time in 1971 Who Were Able or Unable to obtain Permanent Employment in Nursing as of September 30, 1971. Canadian Nurses Association, Ottawa, March 1972, p. 18.

6. Spaulding, W. B., Spitzer, W. O.: Implications of medical manpower trends in Ontario, 1961-1971. Ont. Med. Rev. 39: 527, 1972.

7. Department of National Health and Welfare: National Conference on Assistance to the Physician. Ottawa, April 6-8, 1971.

8. Department of National Health and Welfare: Report of the Committee on Nurse Practitioners (Chairman: Thomas J Boudreau). Ottawa, April 1972, p. 43.

9. Kergin, D. J., Spitzer, W. O.: An Educational Program for Nurse Practitioners. Demonstration Project funded by OHRDP (Award DM36), Ministry of Health, Government of Ontario, Toronto, 1970.

10. Spitzer, W. O., Kergin, D. J.: The nurse practitioner: Calling the spade a spade. Ont. Med. Rev. 38: 166, 1971.

11. Kergin, D. J., Spitzer, W. O.: Final Report—A Pilot Educational Program for Nurse Practitioners. McMaster University, Hamilton, Ont., October 1972.

12. Kergin, D. J., Yoshida, M. A., Tidey, M.: Study of Nurse Activities in Primary Care Settings. McMaster University, Hamilton, Ont., June 1971 (National Health Grant Project No 606-21-48).

13. Department of National Health and Welfare: Report of the Committee on Nurse Practitioners (Chairman: Thomas J Boudreau). Ottawa, April 1972, p. 14.

Nurse Practitioners in Primary Care: The Southern Ontario Randomized Trial*†

W. O. SPITZER, M.D., M.P.H., D. J. Kergin, R.N., Ph.D.,
M. A. YOSHIDA, R.N., M.N., W. A. M. RUSSELL, M.D., C.C.F.P.,
B. C. HACKETT, B.A., AND C. H. GOLDSMITH, Ph.D.

Summary: A group of nurses who formerly had performed office functions received a special university-based educational program designed to prepare them to assume much of primary care management as nurse practitioners. The associated family physicians would shift their role to general supervision and attention to difficult clinical problems. To test this new form of practice, two complementary randomized trials have been conducted in south-central Ontario. The particular trial reported here was intended to assess the influence of the educational program on the changing roles of the professional personnel. The nurses of 14 family medical practices, with the physicians' support and commitment to participation, applied for the new training. Seven applicants were randomly selected to receive the training and their corresponding practices became the experimental group, while the remaining nurses and practices were retained as controls. During the subsequent year of investigation important changes occurred in professional roles of the experimental group. Nurse practitioners spent more time in clinical activities than conventional office nurses. The shift was not at the expense of time devoted to clinical work by physicians. Doctors delegated more professional activities to nurse practitioners than to conventional nurses. Except for remuneration (affected by legal constraints) job satisfaction among experimental physicians and nurses remained high after one year of experience with the new method.

*Originally published as "Nurse practitioners in primary care, III. The southern Ontario randomized trial," in Canadian Medical Association Journal 108: 1005-1016, April 21, 1973. Reprinted by permission.

†This project received support from a grant of the Ontario Medical Foundation and organization support from the College of Family Physicians of Canada. Nurse activity studies were supported, in part, by National Health Grant (Canada) No. 606-21-48.

It is generally acknowledged that doctors in Canada need help to meet the public's demand for ready access to primary medical care. In Ontario, despite a satisfactory overall ratio of one family physician to 1720 persons, access to doctors in various areas is seriously hampered both by population dispersion and by a much lower ratio of physicians to persons.[1]

In recent years the existence of a surplus of nurses in Ontario [2,3] reinforced an emerging multidisciplinary consensus among planners, educators and investigators at McMaster University and at other centres. The belief was that a nurse is the most appropriate professionally trained person to supplement physician care and, in some instances, to replace the doctor.[4,5]

The McMaster University Educational Program for Nurse Practitioners[6,7] was designed to implement this concept. After completion of the program, registered nurses, who had been performing conventional functions in offices of southern Ontario family physicians, have qualified as nurse practitioners or family practice nurses. They then return to the same practices and assume much of the primary care management.

With this new pattern of practice in primary care, the doctors and nurses become co-practitioners. The nurse practitioner assesses patients independently in a large proportion of episodes and is expected to reach a correct action decision. One category of decision for the nurse is referral to the associated physician. With other decisions, the nurse practitioner can provide certain types of health maintenance (such as well-baby care), monitor patient status and therapy for common chronic diseases, and help care for individuals or families with psychosocial problems. In the course of these activities the nurse practitioner makes many minor and occasionally major clinical judgements. The associated physician shifts his (or her) role to one of greater attention to difficult clinical problems and to general supervision of the practice.

Introduction of the nurse as a decision-making co-practitioner is a substantive departure from the conventional mode of clinical management for patients in family medicine. The ultimate effects of this innovation can parallel or transcend the significance of new procedures, new drugs and other new therapeutic regimens.

To be accepted, the new concept required suitable tests of its feasibility. Accordingly, with the support and commitment of physicians and nurses of 16 Ontario private practices, two complementary randomized trials have been conducted in south-central Ontario.

In one trial, designed to assess the effects on patients, the families of two practices were randomly allocated to receive care from the doctor or from the nurse practitioner. We refer to this as "The Burlington Randomized Trial of the Nurse Practitioner." In the second trial, which focuses on the effects upon doctors and nurses, the nurses of 14 practices located in south-central Ontario were randomly assigned to receive nurse practitioner education or to remain in conventional roles. The second project, reported here, has been designated "The Southern Ontario Randomized Trial of the Nurse Practitioner."

GENERAL DESIGN OF THE TRIAL

Only the description of the general design is given in this section. More specific methods are presented with corresponding results in later sections.

Eligibility of Practices to Enter the Trial. The criteria of eligibility for entrance of practices in this trial were delineated in advance and included all of the following:

1. Each medical practitioner was a member of the College of Family Physicians of Canada.

2. The general terms of reference of the nurse practitioners' roles were acceptable to the physician and the nurse in each practice.

3. Each practice agreed to accept the randomization results and to cooperate either as an experiment or control group. (Nurses in the control group were assigned priority for admission to the nurse practitioner course one year after conclusion of the trial.)

4. Each practitioner would submit to all measurements instituted by the research group.

5. Each practice's financial records for the time period of interest would be disclosed to the investigators on request.

6. The practices could not be university- or hospital-affiliated.

7. The practice was located within 50 miles of Hamilton, Ontario, excluding metropolitan Toronto.

The Two Methods of Practice. The contrasting methods to be compared during the 12 months of the trial were as follows: in the conventional practices (the control group), office nurses would provide professional and non-professional assistance to the doctor of each practice in their customary way. Ongoing management of patients would continue to be planned exclusively by the physician based on his (her) clinical judgement. In the nurse practitioner practices (experimental group), the nurses would act as co-practitioners according to ground rules described earlier.

Assignment of Practices. Five months before the trial began, the office nurses of 14 eligible practices had applied for the new training to qualify as nurse practitioners. With random number tables, seven nurses were assigned to receive nurse practitioner training and their corresponding practices became the experimental group. The remaining nurses and practices became the control group (Fig. 1).

Research Questions. The research questions concerning the new method of primary care were in two categories. The first category concerned financial effects upon practices, physicians and nurses. These results, reported elsewhere, showed that family medicine practices with nurse practitioners were not adversely affected in financial performance.[8]

In this report, we focus on the second category of research questions. These were:

1. How is job satisfaction of physicians and nurses affected?

2. Are physicians' and nurses' views of each others' roles changed?

3. How are clinical and nonclinical activities of physicians and nurses altered?

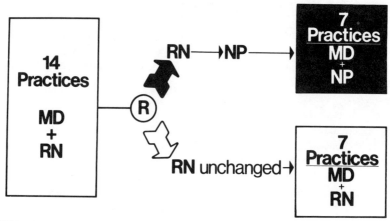

FIGURE 1. Design of the southern Ontario randomized trial of the nurse practitioner. R represents randomization process.

Timing and Implementation of Measurements. The nurses in the experimental practices started their educational program in February 1971 and changed their roles in early April 1971. The trial took place from April 1971 to March 1972. Administration of questionnaires, time and motion studies and observation of practices were undertaken by specially trained interviewers and observers of the Health Sciences Field Survey Unit of McMaster University.

Although the results of such a trial would ordinarily require a set of "before" and "after" assessments, certain logistic difficulties prevented the first set of tests from being performed before the trial began. To allow a true set of "before" measurements would have required an unacceptable postponement of the educational program. Instead, the most feasible approximation of "before" measurements, which were called Time 1 values, was done in April and May as soon as possible after the onset of the trial. Time and motion studies extended into early June. The "after" measurements were completed at Time 2, by March 1972. None of the final measurements were made until at least 10 months had elapsed from the beginning of the trial. Each series of measurements was done simultaneously in the conventional practices and in those with nurse practitioners.

SPECIFIC METHODS AND RESULTS

All 14 practices accepted their random allocations and remained as a part of the study for at least six months. Two practices dropped out before the end of the trial. One experimental practice did so because of professional and financial dissatisfactions. One control practice became university-affiliated. Among the remaining 24 practitioners, compliance to the requirements of the study was nearly perfect. There were minor problems in scheduling some of the measurements.

The individual research questions cited earlier were investigated with the methods and results noted in the sections that follow.

1. How is the job satisfaction of physicians and nurses affected?

Methods: We assessed job satisfaction* of the physicians and nurses using a questionnaire with 67 items that explored: (a) job content, (b) relationships with colleagues, (c) challenge and achievement, (d) available time and energy for the job itself and for other activities, (e) prestige and (f) remuneration. The questionnaire on job satisfaction was adapted from an interview instrument[†] devised for application to professional occupations.[9] A brief excerpt from the questionnaire used, including instructions and examples of some items included, follows:

Instructions:
After each of the following items circle the 'S' if you are satisfied with that item. Circle the 'D' if you are dissatisfied with the item. Circle the '?' if you are not sure. Circle the 'NA' if the item is not present in your job or not appropriate to it. Please mark each item with your present job in mind.

Selected questions:
Job Content
    #16. Committee work required   S ? D NA
    #33. Variety of activities required   S ? D NA
Challenge and Achievement
    #47. Feeling of being needed   S ? D NA
    #56. Chance to evaluate own work   S ? D NA
Remuneration
    #2. Financial security   S ? D NA
    #4. Prospects for future earning   S ? D NA

Since many of the responding practitioners were known to the researchers, an individual not associated with the project or practitioners received and tabulated the instruments. This arrangement was understood by the respondents and allowed them to answer questions without regard to individual relationships.

The maximum possible score (MPS) for all six components of job satisfaction was determined for each individual by adding all the 'S' and 'D' items. The proportion of 'S' items to the total number of 'S' and 'D' items was the score for each individual in the various categories of satisfaction. Maximum possible scores within six categories were then calculated for each individual respondent.

Results: For experimental and control groups the satisfaction scores were expressed as percentages of 'S' items in relation to the aggregate maximum possible scores for the six categories. The scores of physicians are shown in Fig. 2 and of nurses in Fig. 3. With the exception of remuneration, satisfaction scores were high in all components for doctors and nurses of both the experimental and control groups. For remuneration, satisfaction in the experimental group declined in doc-

---

*We have adopted the usual terms used in studies of satisfaction with subjects' work: "professional satisfaction" might have been more appropriate in some ways but might also have been misleading or ambiguous.

†Available from the authors on request.

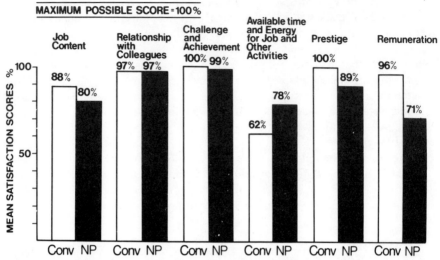

FIGURE 2. Satisfaction of physicians with certain aspects of their work at conclusion of trial (March 1972). Conv = conventional control practices; NP = nurse-practitioner experimental practices.

tors and rose in nurses. Because of the small number of personnel tested, the differences in scores do not attain statistical significance by the usual numerical criteria except in the category of remuneration where the differences are largest and where the probabilities are only borderline.* Nevertheless, we regard the differences as meaningful. They are consistent with the financial concerns expressed by the experimenting physicians in another context,[8] and with the financial dissatisfactions that were partly responsible for the drop-out of one of the experimental practices in this trial. These discontents among doctors probably arise from the current legal restrictions that do not allow charges for the services of an unsupervised nurse practitioner. On the other hand, the higher satisfaction of the nurse practitioners could readily be expected because of their accompanying increase in salary.

2. Are physicians' and nurses' views of each others' roles changed?

Methods: We studied mutual perceptions of the practice pairs using standardized questionnaires. Seven selected situational problems of patient diagnosis and management common in family medical practice were described in detail to each doctor and nurse. For each of the seven clinical problems, the respondents were asked about a variety of different roles or activities.[10] The topics or items were grouped in four categories:

1. Performance of procedural tasks (70 items).
2. Assessment of patients (119).
3. Exercise of clinical judgement (126).
4. Performance of health maintenance functions (217).

*Using the Mann-Whitney U test (corrected for ties), $P = 0.19$ (one-tailed) for doctors and $P = 0.047$ (one-tailed) for nurses. Using Fisher's exact probability test, $P = 0.041$ (one-tailed) against positive association for doctors and $P = 0.064$ (one-tailed) for nurses. We consider that Fisher's test may underestimate the probabilities because the individual observations may not be strictly "independent" in a statistical sense.

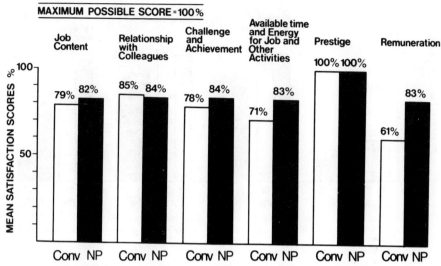

FIGURE 3. Satisfaction of nurses with certain aspects of their work at conclusion of trial (March 1972). Conv = conventional control practices; NP = nurse-practitioner experimental practices.

For each topic, the respondents were asked two questions:
1. Who do you think should perform this role or activity?
2. Who actually does perform the activity in your practice?

When answering, the respondents could choose from four alternatives:
1. Physician only.
2. Nurse only.
3. Interchangeably by M.D. or R.N.
4. Other person.

Scores were calculated separately in each of the four categories of roles or activities for the seven clinical situations. For each category the results were expressed as the percentages assigned to each alternative answer. For example, if there were 40 roles or activities classified in the category "assessment of patients," and a respondent judged 30 of them to be appropriate only to doctors, the score of that respondent would be 75% for opinion about roles appropriate only to doctors in assessment of patients. Similarly, the same respondent could report that the doctor in a given practice in fact performs 36 of the 40 possible roles or activities. The score on actual performance reported would then be 90%. Within a category, e.g., "assessment of patients," the mean of individual respondents' scores was used as the aggregate score for a group such as "control nurses at Time 1" (see Figs. 4 and 5).

Results: In opinions about what work should be done only by nurses, there were no major differences between the experimental and control groups of doctors, either initially or afterward. Similarly, when nurses' views about what activities or roles should be performed only by doctors were elicited, there were no major differences between the groups, initially or afterward. Also, when tabulations were made of items regarded by doctors as proper only for doctors, and by nurses as proper only for nurses, no meaningful contrasts were found.

Some differences did emerge, however, when the physicians identified roles

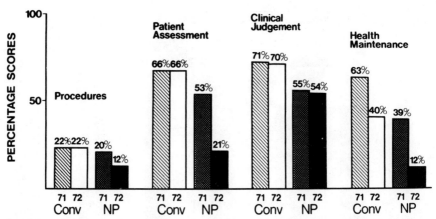

FIGURE 4. Clinical activities performed exclusively by physicians (as reported by physicians). Conv = conventional control practices; NP = nurse-practitioner experimental practices; 71 = Time 1; 72 = Time 2.

and activities they actually performed themselves, to the exclusion of the nurse. The findings are summarized in Fig. 4, which shows the results at the two time periods for physicians in the conventional control (Conv) practices and nurse-practitioner experimental (NP) practices. The height of each column reflects, for all possible activities, the proportion that was performed exclusively by the physicians. As shown in Fig. 4, the percentages of such "exclusively-physician" activities were lower in the NP group as early as Time 1. Later, at Time 2, an even greater reduction for the NP group had taken place in all categories except Clinical Judgement.

The detailed results of the statistical tests for these data are listed in Table I. Differences were considered meaningful in a given category if the P values at Time 2 did not exceed 0.05 and were not higher than 0.1 for differences between Time 1

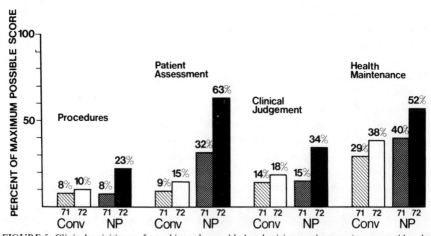

FIGURE 5. Clinical activities performed interchangeably by physicians and nurses (as reported by physicians). Conv = conventional control practices; NP = nurse-practitioner experimental practices; 71 = Time 1; 72 = Time 2.

TABLE I. Clinical activities performed exclusively by physicians*

Probability values:	Comparison of Conv and NP groups†		
	Time 1¶	Time 2‡	Time 1 vs. Time 2‡
Procedures	0.39	0.11	0.23
Patient Assessment	0.042	0.012	0.046
Clinical Judgement	0.016	0.0097	0.16
Health Maintenance	0.042	0.014	0.0065

*Corresponds to Fig. 4 in the text.
†U test (uncorrected) used in column 1 and randomization tests otherwise.
¶Two-tailed probabilities in this column; direction of change not predictable.
‡One-tailed probabilities in these columns; a decline from Time 1 to Time 2 was predicted.

and Time 2.* The noteworthy changes for "activities actually performed exclusively by physicians" are in the categories Patient Assessment and Health Maintenance.

Since the physicians and nurses are assessed as co-practitioners in this study, we were particularly interested in the proportion of activities actually performed interchangeably by either health professional. Fig. 5, constructed in a manner analogous to Fig. 4, shows what was reported as interchangeable by physicians at Time 1 (1971) and Time 2 (1972). Higher proportions of activities or roles were being done interchangeably in experimental practices than in control practices at Time 2. Furthermore, the increases between Time 1 and Time 2 in practices with nurse practitioners were considerably more pronounced than those in conventional practices.

Using the same probability criteria specified for the findings in Fig. 4, the increments for categories Patient Assessment and Clinical Judgement were considered important changes (see Table II).

TABLE II. Clinical activities performed interchangeably by physicians and nurses*

Probability values:	Comparison of Conv and NP groups†		
	Time 1¶	Time 2‡	Time 1 vs. Time 2‡
Procedures	0.31	0.37	0.16
Patient Assessment	0.39	0.0065	0.07
Clinical Judgement	0.18	0.0049	0.095
Health Maintenance	0.39	0.071	0.086

*Corresponds to Fig. 5 in the text.
†U test (uncorrected) in column 1 and randomization tests otherwise.
¶Two-tailed probabilities in this column; direction of change was not predictable.
‡One-tailed probabilities in these columns; an increase from Time 1 to Time 2 was predicted.

*Exact probabilities are given in Tables I, II and III, corresponding to the data displayed in certain figures of the text. Three methods were used to calculate the probabilities: (a) Mann-Whitney U Test,[11] (b) Mann-Whitney U Test with correction for ties,[12] and (c) the Randomization Test (after Pitman).[13] The test yielding the most conservative values (i.e. the highest level of probability values) was chosen for each component of the study. However, the probabilities obtained lead to similar conclusions about the comparisons of interest no matter which of the three statistical tests is employed in the analysis. The reader can select other levels of "statistical significance" for any of the possible comparisons.

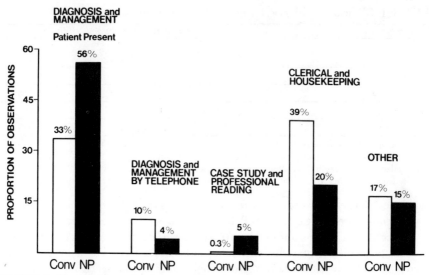

FIGURE 6. Time-motion study of nurses (Time 2, March 1972). Conv = conventional control practices; NO = nurse-practitioner experimental practices.

3. How are clinical and non-clinical activities of physicians and nurses altered?

Methods: To ascertain whether there was any change in the mix of clinical and non-clinical activities undertaken by the co-practitioners in a family practice work-week, we did time and motion studies of nurses and physicians in the experimental and control groups. Each series of time and motion studies of both groups of nurses produced observations every two minutes in a representative sample of 288 half-hour periods during an interval of seven weeks. There were 2160 observations in the experimental groups and 2013 in the controls. For the 12 physicians we cate-gorized and timed all activities in a representative sample of 72 half days during an interval of seven weeks. Because of logistical difficulties, the exact time of sur-veillance was not equal. It was effected for 9202 minutes in the experimental group and only for 7902 minutes in the control group. The inequality in surveillance time did not appear to have any appreciable influence on the results.

Results: Time 1 measurements in this series of assessments were not completed until nearly three months after the trial began. We believe that differences between Time 1 and Time 2 do not reflect shifts in patterns of practice adequately because some of the important changes took place in the first four weeks of the trial. Therefore, only the observations at the conclusion of the trial are shown in Figs. 6 and 7.

Considering the results for nurses first (Fig. 6), diagnosis* and management with the patient present occupied 33% of the conventional nurses' time in contrast to 56% for the nurse practitioners. For diagnosis and management by telephone, the

---

*"Diagnosis" for nurse practitioners is the act of assessing the problem of a patient and reaching a suitable action decision about the problem. Whenever we monitored nurse practitioners' decisions, in over one third of the cases the action decision selected was "refer to associated physician."

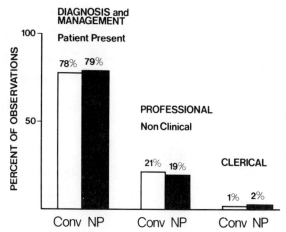

FIGURE 7. Time-motion study of physicians (Time 2, March 1972). Conv = conventional control practices; NP = nurse-practitioner experimental practices.

corresponding values were 10 and 4%. Case study and professional reading during working hours accounted for 0.3% of time in the control group and 5% in the experimental practices. Clerical and housekeeping tasks took nearly twice as much of conventional nurses' time (39%) than of nurse practitioners' time (20%). There was a minor difference for other miscellaneous activities.

To select the categories in which changes were considered important we only took Time 2 differences into account when the P values were less than 0.05. This criterion was met in the category Diagnosis and Management with Patient Present and in Clerical and Housekeeping (Table III).

Although nurse practitioners spent about 50% more time in clinical work and half the time in clerical/housekeeping duties, the shift in time was not at the

TABLE III. Time-motion study of nurses*

Probability values:	Comparison of Conv and NP groups†		
	Time 1 ¶	Time 2 ¶	Time 1 vs. Time 2 ¶
Diagnosis and management (patient present)	0.026	0.042	0.095
Diagnosis and management (by telephone)	0.39	0.48	0.48
Case study and professional reading	0.35	0.48	0.48
Clerical and housekeeping	0.18	0.042	0.064
Other	0.59	0.35	0.38

*Corresponds to Fig. 6 in the text which only shows Time 2.
†U test (uncorrected) employed for all columns.
¶Two-tailed tests used for all columns; direction of change not considered predictable.

expense of time of physicians in clinical activities. Nor did the change noted for nurse practitioners result in a higher proportion of non-clinical or clerical tasks done by the corresponding physicians. As shown in Fig. 7, there were no meaningful or statistically significant* differences between the conventional practices and the practices adopting the new method with respect to activities designated Diagnosis and Management, Professional Non-Clinical and Clerical.

DISCUSSION

It would have been difficult to attain a substantial increase in the level of "job satisfaction" when it was already so high among conventional and experimenting practices. Furthermore, with the small samples available for study, the differences between the groups would have to be substantial before a statistically significant difference would be detectable.

On the other hand, what we consider most important in relation to the research question is that there was no decline in the level of general satisfaction of physicians or nurses in the nurse-practitioner group after one year of experience with the new method except in the area of remuneration. It is noteworthy that despite concern about finances, all the experimenting practices have decided to retain the new approach now that the formal trial is over.

Participation of the experimental group in the nurse-practitioner educational program and in the orientation sessions did not result in differences of opinion between groups about the appropriateness of doctor involvement or nurse involvement in 532 possible activities of family medicine practice. We consider that actual performance of activities is a more reliable indicator of health professionals' perception of roles than their stated views. Compared to control practices a reduction in the proportion of activities carried out exclusively by physicians was reported in the experimental practices. At the same time, more activities were performed interchangeably in the nurse-practitioner group than in the conventional group. Most importantly, the determinations in 1971 and 1972 show the differences became greater with the passage of time with the single exception of activities in the category Clinical Judgement, performed exclusively by physicians.

The assessment of practice activities by objective external observers applying time and motion techniques confirmed what was reported by the practitioners themselves. Compared to conventional office nurses, there were major differences in the patterns of practice of nurses adopting the new role of nurse practitioner. One finding of particular interest to educators of the nurses is that nurse practitioners exhibited a tendency to become self-learners; five months after the conclusion of their formal university course they were observed to spend 5% of working hours in case study and professional reading.

Inferences can only be made about practices of family physicians in Ontario who are members of the College of Family Physicians. These physicians are characterized further by sufficient interest in this new approach so that it is possible

---

*Using Mann-Whitney's U test, the value of P exceeded 0.35 in all categories.

for the nurses associated with them to participate in a demanding post-secondary educational program. It will be many years before nurse practitioners can be trained in our universities and colleges in such numbers that their supply can meet a large demand. It was appropriate therefore, to confine our inquiry to a setting in which the practitioners of nursing and family medicine actively sought to implement the nurse-practitioner role. Within that context, our conclusions are these:

1. Job satisfaction for physicians and nurses does not decline after adoption of the new mode of practice except concerning remuneration among physicians. Physicians and nurse practitioners, having worked as co-practitioners for one year, assessed the concept of provision of primary care by nurse practitioners favourably in all cases.

2. Roles and activities in patient assessment and health maintenance formerly the exclusive domain of physicians are delegated to a greater extent to nurse practitioners than to conventional nurses. Practices with nurse practitioners also exhibit a higher proportion of clinical activities carried out interchangeably by the physician or the nurse.

3. Compared with conventional nurses, nurse practitioners spend about 50% more time in clinical activities and 50% less time in clerical and housekeeping duties.

RESUME*

Resultats d'Essais Effectues dans l'Ontario Meridional

Un groupe d'infirmieres dont la tâche était jusqu'alors purement administrative ont reçu une formation universitaire spéciale conçue pour les préparer à devenir infirmières cliniciennes et à leur permettre d'assumer une grande partie des soins cliniques fondamentaux. Les medécins de famille qui ont participé à ce projet reservaient alors leur rôle à une surveillance générale et à régler les cas cliniques difficiles. Pour évaluer cette nouvelle forme de pratique médicale, il a été décidé d'entreprendre, dans l'Ontario méridional, deux études complémentaires effectuées d'après la méthode du tirage au sort. L'étude qui est rapportée dans le présent article avait pour objet d'évaluer l'influence du nouveau programme de formation sur les nouveaux rôles du personnel paramédical. Les infirmières de 14 bureaux de généralistes, avec l'accord des medecins et l'engagement personnel de ceux-ci à participer au projet, ont sollicité leur inscription. Sept candidates, choisies au hasard, faisaient partie du groupe expérimental, les autres étant considérées comme groupe-temoin. Au cours de l'année qui a suivi le début de l'enquête, d'importants changements ont été notés dans le rôle professionnel des participantes au groupe expérimental. Les infirmières cliniciennes ont évidemment consacré plus de temps à la clinique que les infirmières classiques. Ce changement ne s'est pas fait aux dépens du temps consacré par les médecins au travail clinique. Les médecins ont délégué aux

---

*This summary appears in English at the beginning of this chapter [Ed.].

infirmières cliniciennes une plus grande activité purement professionelle. Sauf en ce qui concerne la rémunération (régie par les contraintes de la loi), les médecins et les infirmières du groupe expérimental étaient très satisfaits de leur nouveau rôle après une annee de fonctionnement.

ACKNOWLEDGMENTS

The authors would like to express appreciation to Dr. Ronald G. McAuley and Miss Norma A. Wylie for their considerable contribution in the earlier formulation and delineation of the problems studied here. Ms. Linda Fischer assisted in certain data gathering and analytical tasks. Miss Eileen Fedor, in collaboration with Audio-Visual Services, McMaster University, prepared the illustrations for the text. Dr. Alvan R. Feinstein was very helpful in reading early drafts of the manuscript and offering constructive criticism. Miss Helen Fulton prepared several drafts of the manuscript. The most essential contribution, however, was made by the members of the College of Family Physicians of Canada and their associated nurses who patiently and cheerfully sustained the investigators' extended surveillance.

REFERENCES

1. Spaulding, W. B., Spitzer, W. O.: Implications of medical manpower trends in Ontario, 1961-1971. Ont. Med. Rev. 39: 527, 1972.
2. Smiley, J. R.: Mobility, Service and Attitudes of Active and Inactive Nurses. A Preliminary Report. Toronto, Research and Planning Branch, Department of Health, Province of Ontario, December 1968, p. 13.
3. Imai, H. R.: Report of a Preliminary Survey to Explore the Nursing Employment Situation in Canada in Terms of the Number of 1971 Graduates of Canadian Schools of Nursing Registered/Licensed for the First Time in 1971 Who Were Able or Unable to obtain Permanent Employment in Nursing as of September 30, 1971. Ottawa, Canadian Nurses Association, March 1972, p. 18.
4. Department of National Health and Welfare: National Conference on Assistance to the Physician. Ottawa, April 6-8, 1971.
5. Proceedings of the Workshop on the Role of Allied Professionals in the Delivery of Primary Health Care. Toronto, College of Family Physicians of Canada, 1971.
6. Kergin, D. J., Spitzer, W. O.: Final Report—A Pilot Educational Program for Nurse Practitioners. McMaster University, Hamilton, Ont., October 1972.
7. Spitzer, W. O., Kergin, D. J.: Nurse practitioners in primary care. I. The McMaster University educational program. Can. Med. Assoc. J. 108: 991, 1973.
8. Spitzer, W. O., Russell, W. A. M., Hackett, B. C.: Financial consequences of hiring a nurse practitioner. Ont. Med. Rev. 40: 96, 1973.

9. Schletzer, V. M.: A Study of the Predictive Effectiveness of the Strong Vocational Interest Blank. Master's thesis, University of Michigan, 1963. Available from University Microfilms, Ann Arbor, Mich.

10. Kergin, D. J., Yoshida, M. A., Tidey, M.: Study of Nurse Activities in Primary Care Settings. McMaster University, Hamilton, Ont., June 1971 (National Health Grant Project No 606-21-48). Document includes examples of interview instruments and a detailed description of the methods used.

11. Mann, H. B., Whitney, D. R.: On a test of whether one of two random variables is stochastically larger than the other. Ann. Math. Stat. 18: 50, 1947.

12. Siegel, S.: Nonparametric Statistics for the Behavioural Sciences. McGraw-Hill, New York, 1956, p. 123.

13. Pitman, E. J. G.: Significance tests which may be applied to samples from any population. J. R. Stat. Soc. 4 (suppl): 119, 1937.

Index